how
to live
when you
could be
dead

*To Hugo, Eloise and Sebastien, for always helping
me to find rebellious hope, even when
I thought I had none left.*

Deborah James

how to live when you could be dead

Vermilion
LONDON

Vermilion, an imprint of Ebury Publishing,
20 Vauxhall Bridge Road,
London SW1V 2SA

Vermilion is part of the Penguin Random House group of companies
whose addresses can be found at global.penguinrandomhouse.com

Penguin
Random House
UK

First published by Vermilion in 2022

www.penguin.co.uk

A CIP catalogue record for this book is available from
the British Library

Hardback ISBN 9781785043598
Trade Paperback ISBN 978178544410

Page design by Nic&Lou and Ed Pickford

Typeset in 11.5/18.2 pt Sabon Next LT Pro by Jouve (UK), Milton Keynes

Printed and bound in Great Britain by Clays Ltd, Elcograf S.p.A.

The authorised representative in the EEA is Penguin Random House
Ireland, Morrison Chambers, 32 Nassau Street, Dublin D02 YH68

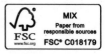

Contents

Foreword by Gaby Roslin   vii

Author's Note   xi

Introduction   1

1 How Hope Can Help You Sleep at Night   8

2 Valuing Today Because Tomorrow Might Not Come   32

3 Something to Aim For   52

4 How I've Kept Going When I Felt Like Stopping   78

5 Fuel the Fire of Failure   98

6 It's Time to Get Gritty   126

7 The Courage to Face Your Fears   152

8 The Healing Power of Laughter   172

9 There's Always Something to Be Grateful For   186

10 Planting Seeds   204

Final Word   213

Resources   219

Foreword

There are times in your life when you meet someone who you know, deep down inside, will make the world a better place. Who will do anything to make you feel happier and more hopeful and fill every day with joy. Deborah is one of those people. Deborah is my friend.

We first met when she was a guest on my radio show. It was clear to me that she had so much to offer, so I asked her if she would like to come on the programme as often as she could. She said that due to her bowel cancer she couldn't commit to anything, as she was living day to day not week to week. But aided by medical treatments, her zest for life and, of course, her fighting spirit, she came back again and again. She phoned in live from her 10ks and marathons, she brought her family along, she joined us at the men's singles final at Wimbledon, but, most importantly, we became friends.

Since then, we have had lots of memorable chats. One that I vividly remember is when she told me how joyous it was for her to have things written in her diary for future dates, as she never imagined she'd be able to do that again.

We've often discussed her treatments, how she's coping, the different things she's being asked to do on TV and radio, but she's mostly wanted to talk about her family. They were, and continue to be, her life. They bring her joy, and she wants to make every single second with them count. For them and for herself. But despite her own problems, she never forgets to ask about my father, who has survived bowel cancer. She always tells me to send him her love.

Deborah loves to dance. She always wanted to be on *Strictly Come Dancing*, but she didn't need to do that to be able to show everyone that music and dance fill her with happiness and help her get through her treatments. It's never just been about her; it's always been about making sure that we all feel that hope and happiness too.

Since being diagnosed, Deborah has been desperate to get the word out about bowel cancer and to tell anyone who will listen that it can affect you at any age. She has openly discussed all the issues surrounding her illness, and she has helped lift some of the taboos around talking about bowel cancer. For far too many years, broadcasters would creep around the subject of bowels and poo and bottoms and symptoms, but not Deborah. She's loud and wants *everyone* to listen and take notice. She's changed awareness. She's changed perceptions. And she's changed people's thoughts and beliefs.

Deborah has also created a cancer community through her social media, which has helped people to feel that they are not alone. That they no longer need to feel so scared. That they can have 'rebellious hope' – and she has been the one holding everyone together.

The last phone call we had was on a beautiful sunny day. We laughed about trying to work out what song we would dance to together in one of our gardens in the sun to embarrass our husbands. She shared with me how ill she really was. I was heartbroken, yet she still made me feel hope. The fact that she has wrung every last ounce out of life is testament to her determination to make every second count – her fashion range, the rose being named after her and, of course, this book are all testament to that.

As someone who adores the bones of this magnificent woman, I cannot tell you how difficult this has been to write, but also what an honour it was to be asked by Deborah to do it. Her laughter and light will live on in us all for a very long time. Let none of us forget to keep hope in our hearts and joy in our days, because that's what she has always wanted. So, Deborah, I promise I will always shout about you from the rooftops. In fact, who needs shouting? I am going to sing loudly and dance around with a huge smile on my face every time I think about my darling, beautiful friend.

Gaby Roslin
June 2022

Author's Note

I started to write this book when I was still feeling relatively healthy and my cancer was progressing slowly. However, as I came to the end of the writing process, my health had deteriorated, and I realised that I probably wouldn't be around to see it published. Rather than go back and change what I've written, I've decided to leave things as they are. This means that, on occasion, what I say comes from the perspective of thinking that I still had a significant amount of time ahead of me. I have done this because I still believe in the lessons I learned and share in this book, even now when I know my time is coming to an end. I am, of course, incredibly sad that I likely won't be around when the book comes out, but I take great comfort in hoping that some of you might find it helpful.

Deborah James
June 2022

introduction

I'm alive when I should be dead. In another movie, I missed the sliding door and departed this wondrous life long ago. Like so many others living with an incurable condition, I've had to learn to live not knowing if I have a tomorrow, because, statistically, I shouldn't have.

At the age of 35, at the tail end of 2016 on a dark, rainy Friday evening just before Christmas, I was blindsided by

The way I approach adversity is my greatest weapon.

a diagnosis of incurable cancer. My change in bowel habits turned out to be a 6.5-cm tumour and, as each month progressed, so too did my cancer. Lung tumours, liver tumours, inoperable tumours – Tumour Whack-a-mole is the worst game ever invented.

I was initially given a less than 8 per cent chance of surviving five years. Writing this book, more than five years later, I have no choice but to live in the now. To value one day at a time, just one, because my tomorrows aren't guaranteed. And neither are yours.

I'm a teacher. I always have been, both in my soul and in my career, which cancer has also taken from me. I've now been out of the classroom for more than five years since that life-changing, world-crumbling diagnosis, but, during that time, I have faced the steepest learning curve of my life. And the drive to learn, to educate, to inspire has become even stronger – it's now just via different platforms: my 'Bowelbabe' blog, national TV appearances, the BBC Radio 5 Live podcast *You, Me and the Big C*, a column in the *Sun*, charity work and, of course, all of the efforts I've made to raise awareness of bowel cancer via my social media channels.

I spend most of my life wanting to escape my incurable bowel cancer, yet there isn't a day that goes by when it's not on my mind. I have loved harder and lost harder than I ever knew possible. I have said goodbye to too many loved ones I've met on this journey – those who wanted just one more second, like Rachael Bland, my wonderful co-host on the podcast who became a true friend and someone I cherished, even though I wish it wasn't cancer that brought us together. It is in their names that I choose to be positive when it would be so easy to give up, and it is because of this that I feel totally alive. I live knowing they would give anything for more life. And so would I.

Every day, I stand at a crossroads: down one path is depression, mind-fuckery, fear of the unknown, heartbreak and mourning – all out of my control; down the other, the one I choose to travel the most (though not always), is positivity and agency. I can't change what's happened or what will happen, but what I am in control of is how I react to my circumstances – that's 100 per cent in my control. Like all of us, I have the ability to make my feelings about my situation, right now, today, anything I want them to be, regardless of the final outcome. The way I approach adversity is my greatest weapon. It's a game changer, and it's all I need – it's all any of us really need.

Each of us faces challenges, large and small, on a daily basis: from relationships ending, moving house or starting new jobs to incurable diagnoses, bereavements or severe traumas. These challenges are, for the most part, out of our control – life seldom unfolds according to a neat and straightforward plan. But what we *can* change is how we approach the difficulties we face, and in this book I'll show you how I have managed not just to cope with adversity but to live with purpose and laughter and a sense of fulfilment that I did not think was possible when I was first diagnosed.

To begin with, we need to stop focusing on 'Why me?' and realise that 'Why not me?' is just as valid a question. How we learn to respond to any given situation empowers us or destroys us – it's how we react to the things on our journey that makes or breaks us. That's why I want to encourage you to question your life as if you didn't have a tomorrow and live it in the way you want today. Being positive isn't keeping me alive, but it's helping me to pick myself up and put myself back together over and over and over again. And the way I have learned to deal with my illness has helped me to live a life full of joy and purpose when I could indeed be dead.

I understand that we are all different, and the things I have found to help me carry on when I am in danger of becoming overwhelmed won't work for everyone, but I hope that sharing some of the more practical things I do might be useful and inspiring for some. I'll explain how instead of admitting defeat in the face of supposedly insurmountable odds, I've embraced positivity. I'll show you how I've harnessed the power of hope even when it seemed like there was nothing to be hopeful about, and how I've learned to value my time and use it more wisely by refining the goals in my life and continuing to create new ones, then implementing the structure and routines to help make them happen. I'll show you how reframing your thoughts can change the prism through which you see things, and that every single thing that happens to you has a lesson in it if you're willing to look for it. I'll demonstrate that grit is a key ingredient of coping with adversity and that we are all more courageous than we realise. Throughout my illness, I've continued to laugh and find the joy in life, and I'll show why this has been so beneficial too. And I'll remind you that, when push comes to shove, it is the little things in life that we are most grateful for.

Whether you've bought this book because you've undergone a traumatic life event, such as an incurable diagnosis, or whether you want to live the life you really want and change the way you respond to challenges, I hope that some of the lessons I've learned will help you to deal with all that life throws at you. I'm living life to the full because I could be dead, and I know you can live your best life too, whatever you might be facing.

The way I have learned to deal with my illness has helped me to live a life full of joy and purpose when I could indeed be dead.

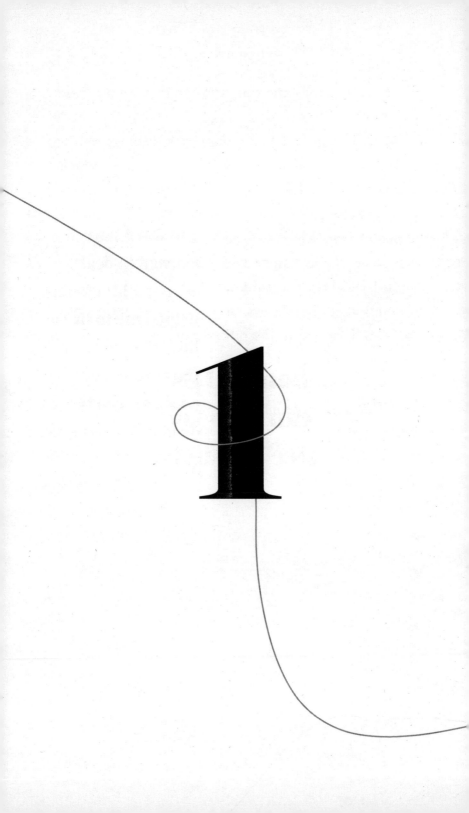

how **hope** can help you sleep at night

'We must accept finite
disappointment, but never
lose infinite hope'

Martin Luther King, Jr

I hope. I hope a lot. I hope cancer won't shorten my life. I hope I continue to be successful and happy in my work. I hope a cure for cancer comes in my lifetime. These are some of my big hopes, but I also hope my kids tidy their rooms and get their homework done. Hope comes in all shapes and sizes, but if you can hold on to it tightly, it will help you to face adversity and even make you more likely to succeed at the things you try. Every time you hit the mat or a bump in the road, hope will help you to pick yourself up again.

Hope is one of the most powerful human emotions we have. When we hear tales of people who have survived being lost in the jungle after a plane crash or adrift in a boat in the middle of the ocean, the survivors often say they never gave up hope – in such extreme situations, it can literally be the difference between living and dying. But it applies to all aspects of life.

When I was first diagnosed in 2016, I was told that I had stage 3 cancer and was given a 64 per cent chance of survival. At the time, it was the worst news I'd ever had, but right now I'd give anything, and I mean anything, for a 64 per cent chance of survival. Then my cancer progressed to stage 4 and was classed as incurable. At this point I didn't see a future, and it took time to regather my thoughts and process the news I had been given. I had to mourn the loss of so much I had taken for granted and somehow pick myself up off the floor and re-evaluate so many things. And one of those was hope – how do you hold on to hope in the face of terrible news and diminishing odds?

But somehow I have managed to remain hopeful, for the most part at least, and I have been kept alive far longer than was expected, in part by drugs that didn't exist when I was first being treated. I just hoped I'd still be here, and I am. I've been incredibly lucky to be able to ride on the coat-tails of science in a way I couldn't have dreamed possible when I was first diagnosed.

I turned to Google when I was initially told I had cancer, hoping to find someone who'd beaten the odds and been cured. I didn't find them, of course, but it didn't stop me from hoping that I might be that person. And it's this kind of rebellious hope that has kept me going. From the beginning, I've flipped the way I view my situation from 'You're going to die' to 'You still have a life to lead. You have a chance of living.' I call it rebellious hope because it goes against what the statistics say about people with my disease. I'm rebelling against expectations of how someone in my position should act, and I'm choosing to remain hopeful despite it perhaps seeming as though there's nothing to be hopeful for. It's my mantra.

I don't claim that it is easy to keep hoping in the face of horrible odds. At those times when life has blindsided you – maybe you, like me, are really unwell, or you have lost your job, or you are going through a difficult break-up – it **Rebellious hope** can often seem like the small **has kept me going.** glimmers of hope that used to come along of their own accord and that you previously relied on to see you through fade and disappear. So how do you regain or hold on to your remaining hope when things seem so bleak? It's incredibly hard, especially against a backdrop of feeling so lost and weak. You feel that there's not a way through and that you're caught in a vicious circle. You feel like you just can't fathom normal life again.

There have been moments when I've been overwhelmed with pain and by what was happening to me. I've found myself thinking at times that life was not worth living any more. I've even said it out loud sometimes, which I know was so hard to hear for the people I loved. But those were fleeting, irrational moments. I didn't really want to die. Dying was the last thing I wanted to do.

It's times like those that have made me realise hope isn't something that just happens to you – it's something you have to actively reach for, to cultivate and to doggedly hang on to when you find even the smallest handhold, especially in the darkest times. When I received my cancer diagnosis, I was really scared, and I was constantly looking for experts – whether that was Macmillan, my GP or an oncologist – to tell me what to do and how best to cope. And, of course, they were full of good advice. But every individual's experience of the illness is unique, and I soon realised that I had to work things out for myself or with the help of my peers. If I was really struggling with the side effects of a treatment, the best approach might not be the stock medical answer; my friend who was also working through a similar problem might have insights that were more relevant to me. Even if I ended up in the same place, there was more value in working out the answer for myself, as I benefitted from full ownership of the solution as well as the knowledge of how to approach similar problems in the future. And being fully invested and believing in the answers I had found for myself only made me feel more hopeful.

I absolutely believe that hope brings strength; the more you have hope, the more likely you are to keep getting back up again when the wind is knocked out of your sails. And it's not just my experience that bears that out; psychologists agree and many scientific studies have demonstrated the important role that hope can play in our lives. The evidence is clear: if you are hopeful, you're more likely to be happy, healthy and successful than if you aren't.

Don't get me wrong, hope in isolation won't make things better. I can spend as long as I like hoping I can run a marathon, but unless I lace up my kicks and train, hoping will get me nowhere. But research studies have shown that people with high levels of hope fare better at times of major life transition and also have better psychological flexibility than their non-hopeful counterparts. In

Finding the answers for myself only made me feel more hopeful.

other words, what it really boils down to is that the more hope you have, the more likely you are to find a solution, to keep going, to get round whatever obstacle is in front of you. Ultimately, hope means staying positive and refusing to let yourself be overwhelmed by darkness and defeat.

'The optimist sees the rose and not its thorns; the pessimist stares at the thorns, oblivious to the rose'

Kahlil Gibran

Throughout my illness, I've thought a lot about whether there is any difference between 'hope' and 'optimism'. They are definitely similar in many ways, and people often use the words interchangeably in everyday life, but they can also be thought of as different traits. On the one hand, optimism is an attitude that things tend to turn out all right in general, even if we have no control over them, whereas hope is the belief that we have a hand in ensuring that things will turn out for the best. So, optimism might mean that you'll always look on the bright side, but hope allows you to find and create a bright side for yourself, even when things are at their most bleak. Although rebellious hope became my mantra, and remaining hopeful has been central to me feeling that I have some control over my response to cancer, I also benefitted at times from a more general sense of optimism and putting my situation in perspective.

A good case in point relates to something in psychology called 'explanatory style'. If you've never heard of this before, don't be put off by the jargon – it simply refers to the way in which people view and interpret the world and their experiences of it, both positive and negative. In other words, it's the stories we tell ourselves to explain what happens to us and why. An optimist doesn't take things personally and tends to think that major events happen because of things outside of their control – if something went wrong, it might be down to bad luck, for example. But they don't see their situation as being permanent or fixed. So if you don't achieve something you had been working towards, it can be the difference between thinking that you didn't practise enough – which is something you can work on – as opposed to a belief that you're just not talented enough. And optimists tend to concentrate on the current circumstances, not leaning towards large-scale, all-pervasive explanations – an optimist who fell victim to a scam would be more likely to come to the conclusion that they had encountered one bad person, whereas a pessimist might surmise that the world is full of dishonest people.

My blog, 'Bowelbabe', became a big part of my own explanatory style. Bowelbabe is my alter ego, in a way, and it allows me to work out a positive but realistic perspective on my situation. I use her to remind myself that cancer isn't personal, that when I hit rock bottom and find myself crying at three in the morning there is a way out, and that when something goes wrong – with my treatment, for example – it's only a small part of my life as a whole. I often get asked if I am faking being optimistic, and I suppose that's one way to think about it: you fake it till you make it. But Bowelbabe is a part of me, and the story I am able to tell myself and others through her is not fake – it's a conscious decision to switch the narrative into something positive and therefore more hopeful.

'If you were allowed one wish for your child, seriously consider wishing him or her optimism. Optimists are normally cheerful and happy, and therefore popular; they are resilient in adapting to failures and hardships, their chances of clinical depression are reduced, their immune system is stronger, they take better care of their health, they feel healthier than others and are in fact likely to live longer'

Daniel Kahneman

When it comes to hope, on the other hand, I'm not referring to an unequivocal belief that you'll succeed – I believe real hope is always grounded in a strong work ethic. You feel like you're going to succeed because you have a plan, a road map and a refusal to yield – and it's these that you can rely on to keep you going. It's about being the force that makes the change. It's not hoping you get the job you applied for because the person who interviews you might like you. It's hoping you get the job you applied for because you prepared so well for the interview and were so focused that you know you're in with a good shot. The right type of hope is dynamic because it gets you moving towards your goal, not just passively waiting for it to come to you.

It's about being the force that makes the change.

This idea of hope as an active process that leads to better outcomes, both when trying to accomplish something in your life and when you are faced with adversity, really speaks to me. Like those plane-crash survivors lost in the jungle, people with hope don't give up and they continue to look for a way out of their predicament, even when things seem to be at their worst.

The great news is that this kind of hope is for everyone. It's a limitless resource and, if you don't already have it, you can definitely get it. Hope doesn't care what your income is or how smart you are, or even what difficulties you are currently facing in your life. It's the same as oxygen – there for all of us all of the time. If you're not a naturally hopeful person or if you've been dealt a hammer blow you don't think you can survive, there are ways you can increase hope in your life and, all things considered, I don't think they are even that hard.

To bring more hope into your life, first try to employ a bit of self-reflection. Think back on the good times, the wins, those occasions when things went right for you. Studies have found that people who are in the habit of reflecting on times when they succeeded and things turned out well report higher levels of happiness and hope than those who don't. It makes sense. Whenever I think about the fact that I have seen five 'last' Christmases come and go, I feel more hopeful that I'll see the next one. I'm reminded that things can and often do go better than expected, despite what I might be going through right now.

Next, there is evidence that prayer and meditation can reinforce our ability to hope. Psychologists have long found that people who do one or the other have higher levels of hope, optimism and self-esteem. It doesn't have to be prayer if you're not religious – it can be as simple as a quiet moment with a cup of tea as you pause and gather your thoughts. Slowing down, taking time and getting yourself into a positive frame of mind is one of the strongest ways you can nurture hope. But you don't even necessarily need to slow down – I found that running gave me the opportunity to be more mindful and in the moment, which is one of the key benefits of prayer and meditation.

It also helps to have faith – and I don't mean in a deity; I mean in yourself. Trust yourself that things can go right, even if they're going wrong right now. Accept that setbacks are part of any journey but not the destination. How can you be your biggest cheerleader? What can you do to remind yourself of how far you've come, what you're good at, how strong you know you can be? It might sound a bit cringe, but practise some exercises where you talk to your reflection in the mirror and repeat phrases that remind you that you've got this, you can do it, you can get through it. Giving myself this kind of pep talk has been really helpful at times when I've been feeling hopeless and, as we'll see later (in Chapter 6), it is also a great way to increase perseverance.

Another good way to increase your hope is to get creative. I don't mean sitting down and drawing or writing poetry – although of course you can do these things if you find that they help you. Studies have found that there's a link between hope and creative thinking – knowing that you can find solutions to problems will keep you positive and hopeful when things get tough. If you've been trying things the same way and they haven't worked out for you, it's easy to get in the frame of mind that you won't be able to find the solution, and that's when hope ebbs away. It's at those times when you need to think outside the box to figure out another route or another way. No matter how bizarre or weird the solution might be, don't discount it. Think, and I mean really think, of the things you could do or how you could come at your 'issue' from another direction. For example, if you're trying to get fitter but not seeing much progress, perhaps it's not your training regime that's the problem – maybe you need to change something in your diet instead. Finding creative solutions to problems also creates a virtuous circle, whereby you feel more hopeful that you'll be able to come up with a solution the next time a problem arises.

This might sound somewhat counter-intuitive, but another way to allow more hope into your life is to think about the worst-case scenario and come up with a strategy to help you face it. Which is not to say that you dwell on the worst thing happening – it's about facing the elephant in the room. What is the thing you're worrying about the most, the thing that is draining your hope? Can you come up with a plan you can trigger if it happens? Of course, the worst thing for me is dying, but I'm not suggesting you come up with a plan of what you would do if you received an incurable cancer diagnosis – worrying about death unnecessarily only leads to anxiety, as you'll see it did for me when you get to Chapter 7. It's more about acknowledging that things sometimes go wrong and trying to anticipate what some of the challenges might be in advance, as it's easier to be hopeful if you feel prepared for the things that life inevitably throws at you. This was definitely an approach that helped me in the classroom – by thinking about what some of the flaws might be in my lesson plans and coming up with some contingencies, I could better prepare for those times when things didn't go quite as I expected.

Holding on to hope is also so much harder if you're exposing your brain to bad news all the time. If you have the news on 24/7 or are addicted to doom scrolling, you'll see a lot of bad in the world. You'll see famine and disease and conflict and disaster and trauma – yes, there's some good news now and again, but predominantly we see what's gone wrong, going wrong or about to go wrong. The world can be a scary place – of course it can. But it is also a beautiful, interesting place full of kind people and fascinating ideas, with lots to feel hopeful about. And don't forget the impact of social media. You need to filter what you're exposing yourself to, limiting the negative but also amplifying the positive – unfollow those toxic accounts, mute the trolls and try to find things to inspire you. Research shows that there's a link between humour and hope, so keep a folder on your laptop or some tabs open on your phone with videos that make you laugh.

Finding stories that give you hope and immersing your-self in them is also extremely powerful. Look for those people who have succeeded 'against all odds', the ones who never gave up, the ones who had hope by the bucket-load. When you can imagine what it's like to feel hope thanks to the inspirational stories of others, you're more likely to feel it yourself and employ the lessons you've learned. Finding a role model is a good way of doing this. For me, I found a dear friend in Rachael Bland. She was diagnosed with breast cancer a month before I was diagnosed with bowel cancer, and we became one another's role models when it came to remaining hopeful and fighting to keep living when we worked together on *You, Me and the Big C*. Our friendship went well beyond us just being colleagues, though, and I am so grateful that I knew her. But it doesn't have to be someone you know personally. Your role model might be a celebrity or a sportsperson – it really doesn't matter as long as they're someone who inspires you as you travel along your own path by exemplifying the positive qualities that you want to emulate, whether that is being a bit braver, grittier or better organised (each of which we'll look at in more depth later).

Hope thrives when it is reflected back at you, so surround yourself with positive people if you can. Eternal pessimists who tell you that you'll never beat your PB, or who constantly express their worries that things won't turn out well, can be hard to be around. We need to be kind if they, too, are going through difficult times, but I think it's often OK to gently remind those people that negativity doesn't get us anywhere and that we need to cultivate hope to move forward. Being around people who are positive and hopeful will mean that those attitudes are more likely to rub off on you. I appreciate that it's not always easy – you can't force the people around you to be more positive if that's not who they are – but there are other ways to get a boost of hope and positivity in your life, like following positive accounts on social media, reading an uplifting novel, joining a group of like-minded individuals, watching your favourite feel-good movie or simply getting outside in nature.

For hope to thrive you need to focus on things that inspire you.

For hope to thrive you need to focus on things that inspire you. For me, it is meeting scientists and oncologists who are developing cutting-edge new treatments for cancer. I'm alive right now because of drugs that didn't exist when I was first diagnosed, and I find that utterly inspiring. My cancer might be incurable, but I know there are inspirational people out there dedicating themselves to prolonging my life and the lives of countless others like me – that's what keeps my hope alive.

* * *

If you try to increase the hope in your life but still feel like you always struggle and can't see a bright side, I've found that it helps to try to reframe the way you see things. Even if it all seems bleak, there will be some brightness. Incurable cancer has brought some of the most wonderful people into my world, from lifelong (or life-short) fellow cancer patients to strangers on the other side of the world. Do I wish I didn't have cancer? Hell yes. Can I reframe it and see the positives it's brought into my life? Yes. Not every minute of every day; not always when I am in pain or when I think about what I will miss when I am gone. But in the main I can.

This might sound like a small thing, but actively changing the language used to refer to my illness has been a really important way of me reframing it. I don't use the word 'terminal' in relation to my cancer – I prefer 'incurable' and very consciously choose to use that word instead. I always correct anybody who introduces me as having 'terminal' bowel cancer because that word focuses on the destination and conjures up the feeling that I'm about to die, whereas 'incurable' makes me feel as though it is a process and that I can plough on. Diabetes is incurable and so is heart disease, and we live with a lot of other incurable ailments that we have learned to control. I hope that one day cancer will just be a disease that we control too. That simple choice of words helps me to reframe my thinking in a positive way and gives me hope, which in turn helps my mental state.

When it comes to hope, this way of framing something is actually far more important than you might think. One of the Nobel Prize-winning psychologist Daniel Kahneman's experiments was to do with the way that people react to a medical prognosis. He found that if you tell someone they have a 90 per cent chance of survival after an operation, they will think very positively about that. But if you tell them they have a 10 per cent chance of dying after an operation, they will think very negatively about that outcome, even though they're actually equivalent statements – they both mean exactly the same thing.

I get a lot of messages from people who are newly diagnosed with cancer who tell me they feel utterly lost and as if there is no hope. They have often just asked, like I did, how long they have left to live. For some, it is a matter of months; for others, it could be years. But either way, their oncologist will have given them an average based on the outcomes for other people who had their type and stage of cancer. Whatever the number is, they can't get out of the loop of thinking about it and, in some ways, of being defined by it. And I'm not saying it's easy to break out of that loop. If you've just walked out of a meeting in which you've been told that, on average, people only live for a couple of years but you'll have some chemo and we'll see what happens, then, faced with this sort of information, it's completely understandable if your first reaction is to feel as though you want to give up, that you've got nothing to live for, that you don't want to go through all of this. The only thing you can do in those circumstances is to reframe the conversation and find examples of hope. And that does not mean simply stepping back and hoping for a bit of luck. There are lots of people who outlive their prognosis and very often it is those who are most positive and engaged in the process in which they now unfortunately find themselves. It is the people who have actively discussed their treatment plans to find one that suits them, or who have asked for a second opinion if necessary, who have more chance of bucking the trend. They question the path they are on rather than passively accepting their fate.

I was involved in setting up a support group for people with bowel cancer on Facebook that is now run by Bowel Cancer UK. When a newly diagnosed person comes on and shares their story, they will be flooded with people saying, 'Oh, don't worry, I was told I was inoperable and I'm still here five years later.' And suddenly they realise that there are examples of people who do survive and recover or who live with the disease in a manageable way for a lot longer than anyone thought possible. And this provides them with hope and something positive to hold on to.

That's partly what motivated me to share my story in the first place. I have a very particular type of bowel cancer. It's pretty rare, with only about 5 per cent of bowel-cancer patients exhibiting this type of mutation, known as a 'BRAF mutation'. The first rule of BRAF club is don't google BRAF. Prior to new targeted therapies being developed, the outcomes were dire for people with the mutation, and I couldn't find a case study world-wide of anybody having lived beyond a couple of years. There was literally no literature anywhere. It's bad enough to be facing a cancer diagnosis at all, let alone to be in that situation with no positive stories to motivate and inspire you. My only option was to reframe the conversation, so I thought: 'OK, I'm just going to have to be my own case study and find a way to outlive my prognosis.'

Hope really is essential in so many ways, adding meaning and purpose to our precious time here on Earth.

Of course, it doesn't always work like that. My body has tried to kill itself on a number of occasions, and hope and a strategic treatment plan can only take you so far. But finding the positive stories so that you can reframe your situation and claim a bit of rebellious hope is the best thing you can do for yourself and for those around you who are on the journey with you.

* * *

My benchmark for hope has changed in the years since I've been diagnosed, which is absolutely fine. Hope isn't static – it changes depending on what you're faced with and how you're coping in the moment. Some of us might just hope we will see another dawn and that tomorrow will be easier than today; some of us hope we can summit Everest in the fastest time possible. I've met some of the most hopeful people I know on cancer wards and during chemotherapy treatments. They might not be hopeful for themselves or their own outcomes, but at the very least they remain hopeful for those they'll leave behind.

The truth is, hope really is essential in so many ways, adding meaning and purpose to our precious time here on Earth. Without it, our ability to deal with adversity would be greatly reduced and our lives as a whole diminished. Whatever your situation, I believe you need to hold on to hope and nurture it when you find it. And when you are facing something frightening, it's absolutely vital. Without hope, I'd literally be a quivering mess of tears in a puddle on the floor. So no matter what you might be facing, always remember that hope can show you a way through.

'To live without hope is to cease to live'

Fyodor Dostoyevsky

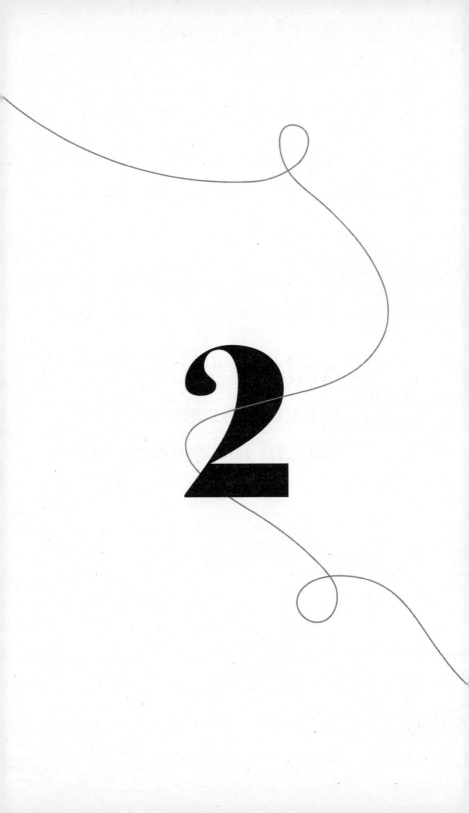

valuing today
because tomorrow
might not come

'Do not squander time, for that's the stuff that life is made of'

Benjamin Franklin

When I was a teacher, we used to take the sixth-formers away every year on a retreat. I'd run workshops with the kids – well, they were 17 and 18 years old, so they were actually young adults – and I'd read them a piece by a French writer called Marc Levy about time and how we use it. I suppose it is a bit cheesy in some ways, but it really pulled my strings when I first heard it as a teenager. It asks the reader to imagine that they have a bank account that is credited with $86,400 every day, but every evening anything that isn't used is lost, only to be topped up again with the same amount the next morning. If you had such an account, you'd spend every dollar, wouldn't you? Levy goes on to explain that we do have such a bank account, but that every morning we receive 86,400 seconds, and the time that we don't use is lost for ever:

If you fail to use the day's deposits, the loss is yours. There is no going back. There is no drawing against the 'tomorrow'.

The point the piece is making is that we must make the most of the time we have every day because we can't get back those seconds, minutes or hours once they are gone.

I'd then give each student a notebook and ask them to write down what they were going to do with their time. It was a means of making them think about time and whether they used it effectively – well, as far as is possible with young people who are inclined to view time as an infinite resource! I know I waste time, going down rabbit holes on social media, for example. I think we all do. So I wanted the students to recognise this and realise that valuing time and using it constructively is a challenge and something we have to actively consider.

We all know that time is precious. We all know, rationally speaking, that it will eventually be taken from us, and yet we somehow don't really think it's ever going to end – many of us don't truly get past our teenage perception of infinite time. We think that we can put things off to another day or that we can buy more time. But sometimes there is no tomorrow. Each of us has 86,400 seconds every day, and we assume they will keep on coming day after day, for many, many years – and for millions of people they do. But for me and others like me they will run out so much sooner than we ever thought they would. I don't know when that will happen, so I have to live in the moment and use my positivity every single day to find hope and contentment, even in my darkest times.

I was privileged to interview Kathryn Mannix, the inspirational palliative care nurse and author, for an episode of *You, Me and the Big C*. She said that we always assume that there is more time, but in fact there are two days in our lives when we won't see the full 24 hours: the day that we were born and the day that we die. And I remember thinking at the time that it was quite a stark reminder that many of us assume the clock will always tick 24 hours of the day for us, but actually our time will run out.

Even after I discovered I had cancer, it took a little while for this message to sink in. Not long after being diagnosed, I came across someone on Twitter who found out at around the same time as I did that he had bowel cancer too. It was the first time I'd really used social media, because teachers tend to steer well clear in case their students get wind of something they shouldn't. I didn't really know how to use it at first, so I'm not sure how I discovered him, but he was talking about bowel cancer. He was about my age, and he had two really young kids. I messaged him to say hi and that it looked like we were going through the same thing. We compared notes about how many lymph nodes we had infected with cancer and what our operations had been like. And then something happened that came as a shock to me at the time – he never left hospital. He told me in his messages that he was really not well, that his cancer was rapidly progressing and that he was being moved to a hospice.

We can't take our time for granted.

Eight weeks later, he died. He'd been diagnosed with cancer and two months after that he was dead. I remember thinking, 'Oh my God, people actually die.'

I was completely naive. I knew I had cancer, and I knew it was serious. There were some really scary statistics when it came to people in my position. And, in fact, at that time, I was actually only days away from being told I had stage 4 cancer, which brings with it even more dire statistics about survival rates. But, at that time, following a successful operation and in light of the number of infected lymph nodes that I had, I'd been told that I had maybe a 64 per cent chance of survival. And yet my Twitter friend had been given a better prognosis, with fewer infected lymph nodes than me, and he had died. I remember thinking, 'This is a vicious disease; anything can happen.' It was my first experience of speaking to somebody online and then saying goodbye to them. It made me realise that this was the world I now lived in, and it motivated me to make the most of the time I had left, because I now knew that I was a ticking time bomb. It was like a slap in the face: 'OK, I'm not dead yet, but this could happen really quickly. It's very real. So, what do I do? Do I sit and cry or do I get up and face this head-on?' And that became something that motivated me.

Then, when the medical options ran out for me in May 2022, I was blindsided by the realisation that, even though I had been living with an incurable cancer diagnosis for more than five years at that point, my time was up; maybe I didn't have ten more minutes or the next hour of my life. It is a heartbreaking realisation that you can't just say, 'I'm going to do that tomorrow' or 'I'm going to do that next year', and a stark reminder that we can't take our time for granted.

* * *

When I was juggling my work as a teacher with my hectic home life, I was always busy and never thought there were enough hours in the day. And I wasn't alone. Despite our free time having increased since the 1960s, by as much as five to seven hours a week by some measures, according to one study, 34 per cent of us feel rushed all the time, 61 per cent of us don't think we have any excess time and 40 per cent of us think a lack of time is a bigger problem than a lack of money. There is a tendency for us to think that the solution to this problem is more time or better time management. And while many of us could certainly use our time more effectively, the truth is that neither of these things is the real answer to easing the pressures on our time. I think that what really matters to our well-being is how we perceive time.

Psychologists have identified five different ways that individuals generally think about time:

1. Future-oriented
2. Present-hedonistic
3. Present-fatalistic
4. Past-positive
5. Past-negative

People who are **future-oriented** plan ahead and work towards long-term goals. They also tend to delay gratification, thinking that the pay-off will be better if they wait. Overall, future-oriented people tend to be healthier and more successful in their careers, but they can also be workaholics who neglect their relationships and unnecessarily deny themselves good things that they will enjoy in the present.

Present-hedonistic people are the polar opposite, living for the moment and seeking out thrills and excitement. They don't really think about the consequences of their actions, which can lead to unnecessary risk-taking. The majority of children have this time perspective to begin with, but it fades with age in most people. However, those who maintain a present-hedonistic outlook into adulthood can be more likely to succumb to addiction. On the plus side, people with this perspective are open to new experiences and can experience real highs, although these can be followed by steep comedowns.

Those who tend towards a **present-fatalistic** time perspective also live in the moment but feel helpless and hopeless, often believing that forces outside their control are shaping their lives. This negative mindset doesn't have a lot going for it, although a dose of scepticism and a sense of restraint, which can also be features of this perspective, can sometimes be healthy.

Past-negative is a similarly damaging time perspective. People who tend towards this outlook can find themselves haunted by the past, always focusing on bad experiences and what went wrong.

Past-positive people, on the other hand, look at the past with affection, which makes them more likely to value their long-term friends and family. People with this outlook tend to have the highest self-esteem out of the five types, and they also enjoy more success and satisfaction in their personal lives. Too much sentimentality about or nostalgia for the past, however, can result in excessive conservatism and caution, leading to people rejecting anything new and unfamiliar, and a desire to maintain the status quo, even if it has become damaging to them.

Do any of these sound like you? Although our time perspectives can change over the course of our lives, one tends to be dominant at any given time, and they can persist over long periods. In retrospect, I can see that I had pretty clearly defined time perspectives at various points in my life. When I was a teenager and prior to beginning my career in teaching, I was very much a present-hedonist whose main aim in life was to have fun. Then, when I started work as a teacher and realised I'd found a job I loved, I threw myself into it and had a much more future-oriented perspective – it would probably be fair to say that I was a bit of a workaholic and sometimes neglected my relationships. It wasn't until I was diagnosed with cancer that my outlook shifted to prioritise a past-positive perspective, and I realised that the most important thing in my life was the people I loved.

While there are obviously upsides to positive thoughts about the past, present and future, there are also costs to each perspective. That is why it is important to really consider how you think about time and your relationship with it, and strive for a more balanced approach. If you work long hours chasing your next promotion, like I used to do, you should take a break now and again and spend some time with your loved ones. If you blow all your money as soon as you get paid on going out and having fun, think about saving some for a rainy day. And if you have an overly romantic view of the past, perhaps try to open yourself up to meeting new people and experiencing something different – you will probably surprise yourself with how much you enjoy a change from the norm. The key is to be flexible and adopt a time perspective appropriate to the situation. If you can do this, you increase your chances of creating a healthy work–life balance and improving your well-being overall.

Of course, 'balance' is subjective – what works for one person won't necessarily work for the next. Some people really benefit from a clear division between work and home, whereas someone else might get more stressed out if they don't check their work emails at the weekend. Find what works for you, and take a moment every now and again to check if one time perspective is dominating your life too much.

> **I realised that the most important thing in my life was the people I loved.**

* * *

I don't have the luxury of time I thought I had in 2016, and that lack of time speaks to every single one of the goals I make for myself (more of which in the next chapter) and how I spend my days. Think about your daily behaviours and what you'd change if your tomorrows were limited. Perhaps you are one of those people who doesn't like to think too much about how many tomor-rows you might have (and I don't blame you – it's not a pleasant thing to contemplate). But if you put off moving towards what you want or doing the things that are truly meaningful to you because you think you have all the time in the world, you're living like you'll live for ever, and that's not a possibility for any of us.

As I've mentioned, Rachael Bland and I were diag-nosed at the same time. We broadcast together and rode the highs and lows of our joint diagnoses on a cancer rollercoaster, including the darkness of the 3am fear. But her fear became her reality sooner than mine. On paper, she should still be here now, and I should be the one who's gone. Statistics told her that she had an 80 per cent chance of a future, while I only had an 8 per cent chance of living for more than five years.

Sadly, over time, I've lost lots of friends to cancer, some of them really, really close friends. I think social media is amazing, but I've learned to be a bit careful about the relationships I create online. I know now that there are thousands of people living with bowel cancer and dying from bowel cancer. And not just bowel cancer – all types of cancer. The opportunity social media presents to fill your feed only with stories of cancer is potentially quite dangerous, as you can live in an incredibly dark world if you're not careful. That's why I seek out the inspirational and positive online as much as possible.

However, at the same time, my motivation for living became very much linked to the realisation that there are too many people who I've met or connected with on social media who just wanted one more day. But none of us know exactly how much time we have left. Nothing is set in stone and nothing in life is predictable.

This is a realisation that usually comes with the wisdom of age. As we grow older, we become more aware of our mortality, and our outlook on life changes as a result. When we are infants, the passage of time since our birth is a useful way of measuring our physical and psychological development, from when we are likely to say our first words to when we will have the coordination and strength to take our first steps. As we move through childhood and into adulthood, age becomes a less precise measurement of what we are capable of, because there are a huge range of variables that determine how we develop as people. Age is still a rough indicator of general life experience, but increasingly it doesn't really tell you much beyond that.

Stanford psychologist Laura Carstensen has shown that our perception of how much time we have left is a more reliable indicator of how we behave and what we prioritise than simply how old we are. When we are younger, most of us have the sense that our lives will be in the region of the average – in the UK, this is just over 81 years old. This sense of how much time we have left has a profound effect on the way in which we approach life. There are obviously exceptions at both ends of the spectrum, but young people tend not to think too much about time running out and, as a result, tend to be more open to new experiences, meeting lots of new people and acquiring more knowledge, whereas older people are more likely to prioritise their well-being and deeper, more meaningful relationships and pursuits. This theory goes some way to explaining why young and old people report roughly the same levels of general happiness. We may do less when we are older and have a smaller social network, but we take more satisfaction from those things than a busy young person who is intent on learning new things and broadening their horizons.

Although this process happens naturally as we grow older, Carstensen has shown that the same shift in priorities can happen regardless of age – if we become more aware of the fragility of life. My priorities changed completely after cancer – the desire to live well and to forge even more meaningful relationships with the people I love was what mattered to me most. But I wish it hadn't taken this catastrophic situation for me to adopt this perspective. If you can, regularly remind yourself that time is finite and you never know what's round the corner. The realisation that your time is precious is fundamental to living a fuller and more meaningful life now.

We can be blindsided by awful, or simply unexpected, things at all stages of our lives – losing a home or a job, an incurable diagnosis, the loss of a loved one. The only thing we can do when life sends us into a spin is to teach ourselves how to ride it – to change, adapt, survive and even smile in the darkness.

While my cancer diagnosis was a seismic shift for me, it's not the only one I've experienced. Finding out I was pregnant at 24 with my now-teenage son Hugo, although it turned out to be one of the best things that ever happened to me, made the wheels come off my wagon, as it was never my plan to become a mother at that age. So did saying goodbye to my 17-year-old cousin when she died in a car accident 20 years ago. So, too, did Covid-19, but I came through each a stronger person and that's down to the questions I asked myself and the sacrifices and choices I made and continue to make along the way.

As my illness has progressed, I've always hoped that a couple of months might turn into six months of life, and then you never know. In January 2022, I didn't think I would be alive come May, but I was, albeit most of it was spent in a hospital room. During that period, I had to learn to live in the snippets of time that I had left and not just wait to die. And that was so hard because you need to witness life in order to have the energy to want to live it – being trapped in a hospital room for weeks on end really saps your morale and zest for living. But I always try to create a virtuous rather than a downward cycle, and that includes valuing the time I have left, down to the very last days, minutes and seconds.

This is why I've tried so hard to make lasting memories since becoming ill and especially as it became clear that my time was running out. I've done lots of amazing things

I had to learn to live in the snippets of time that I had left and not just wait to die.

since being diagnosed, of course, from going on TV, writing my column and doing the podcast to running the London Marathon and visiting the Chelsea Flower Show to see a rose named in my honour, but it is the memories I've made with my friends and family that mean the most to me. I've made new bonds with people like Rachael Bland and Gaby Roslin, and I've deepened my relationships with my existing friends.

But there is one memory from when I transferred to hospice care at my parents' home that stands out in particular. After I'd been there for about a month, I was sleeping more and more, and my energy levels were such that I couldn't really leave the house or even get out of bed all that much. I was feeling really down about it, so my sister Sarah suggested we have a family sleepover. I wasn't sure if I was up for it, as I was feeling so tired and emotional, but when they brought me into the room in my wheelchair and I saw the tepees and the fairy lights and the decorations, I cried good tears. The girls in the family (and my brother Ben, who was an honorary girl for the evening) snuggled into the cushions and blankets with me and watched *Cinderella*, and I felt like I was five years old again. It brought such a smile to my face – Cheshire cat level – and I knew that it was a memory that we would all cherish, especially my mum, my brother and sister, and my daughter Eloise. The next day I slept, but with another memory and a smile.

Making memories like this one to get you through the hard times, and for those you leave behind, is, in my opinion, something we should all devote more time to whenever we can. It is the best way I know of making the most of every day.

* * *

Each December since I can remember, I wrote a list of all the personal things I'd achieved that year and what I wanted to achieve still. Year on year, without fail, it included:

- Run the London Marathon.
- Buy a new house (or something else that I couldn't currently afford).

- Something involving DIY that was unlikely to ever materialise.
- Go to the gym five times per week.
- Save X amount of money by the end of the year.
- Go on holiday to a faraway location.
- Take up a hobby that was never going to happen – whether that was becoming good at cooking, or learning how to sew, or taking ballroom dancing lessons or doing a photography class.

Despite writing them down, I never really achieved any of these things (except for running the London Marathon) because I didn't have a plan for how I'd achieve them, and I didn't set myself a time frame (something we'll talk about more in the next chapter). There was no real urgency because time seemed open-ended – everything on the list could be put off until next year.

My biggest motivation has been making the most of the time I have.

Some of those 86,400 seconds you get every day need to be spent on moving closer to what you want from life, because once they're gone, they won't come back. Just as the piece of writing I quoted from Marc Levy at the beginning of this chapter says, you can't 'bank' the time you're given in a day and carry it over to the next one, so you might as well start using your days better. I really believe that you must remind yourself to look to the future with hope and optimism, but that it is equally important to value the here and now. You can value the past, live in the moment when you want to have fun and plan for the future in equal amounts, depending on your changing circumstances and shifting priorities, as long as you remain conscious of valuing your time and realise just how precious it is.

Since my diagnosis, my biggest motivation has been making the most of the time I have. I *have* to invest those seconds into what I want most – to live well – because I have no idea when the account will close. I invest in health and happiness and positivity because it's vital that I make the most of every day, for me and the people I love.

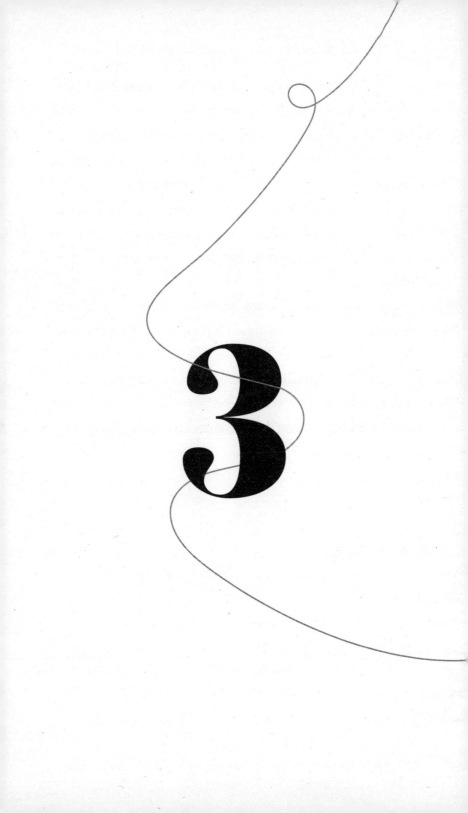

something to
aim for

> '**If you want to be happy, set a goal that commands your thoughts, liberates your energy and inspires your hopes**'
>
> Andrew Carnegie

During the last term of secondary school in 1996, my friends and I recorded a video on a camcorder borrowed from one of our parents. Our giddy teenage aim was to state our plans and goals, then watch it back at 30 and see how close we were to what our 16-year-old selves had thought of as constituting success and happiness.

My goal in life at 16 was to marry my then-boyfriend, Paul. I was going to have three children and life would just be 'fine'. That was it. The sum of my desires and goals was marriage, children and a 'fine' life. Nothing at all relating to work, a career, study, travel or venturing beyond my own little corner of the world.

Why were my goals so limited? Probably because my parents had done a fantastic job of shielding me from the big, bad world. I'd experienced little to no hardship. I hadn't encountered sadness or trauma. My most pressing worry was boys and making sure I proved my careers adviser wrong when she said that I shouldn't aim to go to university. I didn't form more rounded goals because I hadn't experienced very much.

My kids, however, have spent a significant portion of their lives with me having cancer. My teenage daughter Eloise's goals are varied and plentiful. She wants to be a fashion designer, artist, presenter, chef, interior designer and party planner. If I ask where boyfriends or children figure in her goals, she wrinkles up her beautiful face at me like I'm speaking another

I wish I'd considered that things could be taken away from me, that the future isn't certain for any of us.

language. I admire her ambition to achieve many different things and wish she'd been my friend when I was a hapless teen thinking about my future. Eloise is hungry for experience and living life to the full because she knows things don't always work out like you plan them. She's hyper aware that life changes and can be cut short, and her passion for living reflects that.

Looking back at my naive younger self, I wish I'd been a bit more ambitious with my hopes and dreams. I wish I'd considered some goals that would have pushed me or been a challenge to reach. I wish I'd considered – even for a nanosecond – that things could be taken away from me, that the future isn't certain for any of us.

I was in my twenties when I discovered my goal to be an educator. Because I never really took school all that seriously, it might seem a bit ironic that teaching became my vocation, but I knew almost immediately that it was the right career for me. The opportunity to shape the lives of my students, some of whom were still trying to find their way in life, as I was at their age, was a real privilege and something I threw myself into. I wanted to change the world, one pupil at a time. I wanted to prove to young people that they could reach for the stars.

With such a strong sense of purpose in place, and increasing ambition to further my teaching career, I became very good at strategic planning, breaking down tasks into achievable parts, making a five-year development plan and setting milestones. I went from being a sheltered 16-year-old with a rather limited view of the world to a person who always had to have a plan, in my personal life as well as at work. I became a deputy head by the age of 30, and I actually wanted to be the youngest head in the country, before I realised someone had beaten me to it. Instead, I decided that I wanted to be a head by the time I was 35, which is still quite young by today's standards, even though the average age is trending downwards. In retrospect, I realise that I possibly had too much structure in my life at times, as it meant that I sometimes didn't know how to go off-piste, and everything was planned a year in advance.

As I rapidly worked my way towards being a head teacher before the age of 40, the vital benefits of goal-setting became increasingly apparent, when it came to both my own aspirations and those of the kids I was teaching. Then my cancer diagnosis came along and, unsurprisingly, I was pretty much blindsided. I thought I had a great positive mindset, but I wasn't prepared for such a big and unexpected challenge. I'd become quite good at strategic planning and being able to say, 'Right, this is what I'm going to do.' I had worked hard on my professional goals because I loved my job and wanted to excel at it. But it now looked like my immediate career plans at best and my very future at worst were to be taken from me.

When I realised not long after being diagnosed that my treatment plan and teaching weren't going to be compatible and that I therefore couldn't have the career I'd planned so meticulously and worked so hard for, it was incredibly challenging. Not only was I mourning the fact that I had cancer, I was mourning the loss of my career and a big part of the means by which I defined my worth. And what I didn't realise at first was that it wasn't only my career I was losing – it was the community that teaching gave me as well. I obviously had many friends outside of teaching, but that big support network that you get when you see people every single day in an environment that you know, that you feel supported in, that is your home from home, is almost as big a loss.

At first, I plummeted to the depths of hell and didn't really know how to do anything, how to process what was happening to me. I felt like I was losing so much of what I valued in my life: my job, my youth and my health. I was so low that I just couldn't get out of bed. About three months after my initial diagnosis, my mum and a very good friend of mine said to me that I needed to get up because I really smelled. They said I should get in the shower and then I could go back to bed if I really wanted to – I just needed to move.

I had no idea how I was going to cope with the new realities of my situation. I was in a state of utter disbelief at first and felt totally lost. It absolutely wasn't a case of saying, 'Oh, yes, I know, I'm going to be strong and positive and put all these strategies in place.' I was adrift, and I had to find a fresh sense of purpose and new goals – but first I just had to find a way to get out of bed, gather my thoughts and get through each day.

Not only was I mourning the fact that I had cancer, I was mourning the loss of my career and a big part of the means by which I defined my worth.

What would turn out to be key for me in being able to stay positive in the face of cancer was finding renewed purpose. People often say, 'Well, you've got kids. You've got purpose.' Of course my kids give my life purpose – they mean everything to me – but I've always been somebody who has been career-driven, and I need something else too. I pour a huge amount of my energy and emotion into looking after my kids, which makes it all the more heart-breaking that cancer will one day rob me of time with them, but I also need something that's just mine. It doesn't mean that I love them less. Plus, they are getting older and need me less than they used to, or at least they need me in a different way. Finding a purpose again was, therefore, about finding the thing in my life that would motivate me to keep going alongside what I get from my family.

At first, I didn't really know what that might look like for me, but it ultimately became apparent that it was sharing my story. I'd never really written much in my life before then, but that's when I decided I would start my 'Bowelbabe' blog. This would also help give me structure, which is something I have always needed, as I decided that I was going to write it once a week. I suppose part of me thought that was how I was going to get through every Monday: 'What am I going to do on a Monday? I'm going to write a blog. That's my Monday sorted. Great.' It was a way of finding purpose and helping me to get back on my feet.

From the blog, things just kind of escalated and new opportunities presented themselves and I jumped on them.

It was a way of filling the massive void in my life once teaching – something I'd worked hard at for many years – was essentially ripped away from me. And it gave me a purpose beyond just staying alive, because it can become quite soul-destroying if the only thing you can think about is cancer. It was through this that I ended up writing a column for the *Sun*, co-hosting the podcast *You, Me and the Big C* with Rachael Bland and Lauren Mahon, and publishing my first book (*F*** You Cancer*) – things that I would never have thought possible when I was a teacher.

Finding your why, like I did, will help you take control of the steering wheel, turn it towards the right road and make sure you're heading in the direction of what you want in life. Having purpose will help you to choose your goals, which in turn can function to reinforce the things that are most important to you and help to define who you are, adding meaning to your life. In fact, the more closely aligned your goals are to the things that matter to you most, the more likely you are to commit to them, and the more satisfaction you will take from them. This is why it is important to set goals that mean something to you, as well as ones that you actually have a chance of achieving.

* * *

While I'm not making any decade-long plans any time soon, once I got my feet back on the ground after my diagnosis I did start to make goals that would take longer to achieve and weren't just focused on getting through my treatment and staying alive: some big and some small. For example, I've nailed making a mean Yorkshire pudding, and I decided I was going to sort out my wardrobe –

'Bowelbabe' was a way of finding purpose.

although, to be honest, that one hasn't gone quite so well! An important one I made shortly after I was diagnosed was to be more present in the moment. I'm now present in a way I wasn't before cancer. I decided I wanted that to be one of my goals, realised I had to dedicate time to it and started working on it immediately – and I've worked on it every day since then.

A small example of being more present meant not taking my mobile phone to the dinner table or scrolling through my social media feeds while watching a movie with the kids. More generally, it meant prioritising my family in a way that I didn't when I was a busy career mum rushing around trying to squeeze everything into my jam-packed schedule. My illness has taken away a lot of things from me, but I can now say with absolute honesty that it's given me a lot too, and, strange as it may sound, I'm grateful to it in some ways. Being more present is one of those things.

Of course, I'd give a lot of this up just to have a long-term future again. I'd do just about anything to go back to my goal of being a head teacher and making my mark on the education system in this country. But that goal is gone, so I've had to adjust and make new plans, find new ambitions. It's not been easy, but I have (for the most part) been able to reframe my perception of my situation and see my cancer diagnosis as a chance to do other things. I've looked for opportunities and potential in place of failure and loss, and made the most of the life I still have.

Continuing to form goals in the face of incurable cancer has allowed me to carry on with purpose and motivation, making me feel as though I am in charge of my situation rather than sitting back and waiting for the inevitable, and I believe that goal-setting is something that can help all of us, no matter where we are in our lives right now or what challenges we might be facing.

I realise that I may well be preaching to the converted, and most of us set goals all the time, but I can't emphasise how vital they have been to me, especially since being diagnosed. And that is so important to stress: goals are arguably even more important when the shit hits the fan and things aren't going to plan.

It is at those times that the real benefits of goal-setting shine through. For one thing, having something to aim for is a brilliant way to stay motivated, maintain momentum when things are difficult and keep a positive outlook about the future. If all I had to aim for was the end of my life, it would be so dispiriting; even with my health at its worst, I still try to stay engaged and make plans, whether that is keeping up to date with all of my projects to raise awareness of bowel cancer or helping my brother Ben and his girlfriend Ashley arrange their wedding after he *finally* got round to proposing to her (if you ever followed my podcasts, you'll know that brother banter featured highly!).

My goals provide me with a road map through the hard times, helping me to move forward, and they play a significant role in defining my values and beliefs and investing my life with meaning. When I've been at rock bottom, stuck in a hospital bed for weeks on end, having something to work towards has had such a restorative effect. A good case in point is the clothing line that I launched with the fashion brand In The Style. Seeing that come to fruition in May 2022, first with the release of my 'Rebellious Hope' T-shirts and then with the whole collection – featuring a variety of dresses, skirts, tops and more in beautiful prints and colours that represent British summertime – gave me a huge boost. I thoroughly enjoyed being involved in every step, from choosing the fabrics, prints and designs to ensuring that each item was something everyone would feel amazing in. To see one of your goals real-ised, after all of the planning and hard work that has gone into it, is like a shot of adrenalin to your self-confidence.

Having goals also helps you to prioritise, both in terms of identifying the things that are important to you and also more practically by allowing you to work out what needs to be tackled first. And there are other practical benefits. You are more likely to put effort into something if you are working towards a clearly defined goal, and to keep going if and when you encounter challenges. Goals also make you accountable, most importantly to yourself. Whenever another year passed without me achieving one of my goals, the person I was mainly letting down was myself. This doesn't matter so much if the goal is to have a tidy wardrobe, but if the goal is meaningful to you and you haven't put in the effort to try to make it happen, it's important to take stock and assess what you need to do differently.

If you've recently been through a life-changing event, it might feel quite natural to take stock and look at where you've come from and where you're going. After all, one of

My goals provide me with a road map through the hard times.

the few good things about 'life shocks' is that they can jolt you out of your everyday routine and force you to step back and consider the bigger picture. The death of a loved one, the loss of a job or a terrible health diagnosis can all be the impetus for us to evaluate our journeys so far and maybe change direction. But, at the same time, I don't believe that it should take a personal catastrophe to re-evaluate your goals. Maybe you've reached a milestone birthday, or a friend has changed an important aspect of their life and you've seen the results. Maybe it's simply because today is Tuesday and you've started to read this book.

Whatever the impetus, it's always worthwhile asking yourself what your goals are in life. My goals change, but, in essence, because of my circumstances, my main goal is that I want to live. It's not that simple, though – no goal is. In reality, I want more than that – I want to live well. And that's the same for all of us, right? No one aspires to just get through each day, even if sometimes when life is tough that is realistically all we can manage for a short time. We want to live a life that makes us feel happy and fulfilled. But what does that look like? What does 'living well' mean to you?

Goal-setting is pointless if the goals we've picked drive us in a direction we don't wish to travel, or if they don't drive us at all, like my goals as a 16-year-old didn't drive me. Similarly, if your current goals don't inspire you, they might be the wrong ones for you. For the most part, goals should have meaning to them, even if that meaning is only relevant to you. It is also worth saying that goal-setting in some circumstances can have disadvantages.

For example, if failure to perform a goal brings with it the threat of punishment or some other negative consequence. If you are asked to adopt a goal by someone else – a boss, say – that is impossible to achieve, it can cause you real stress and anxiety. That is why it is important to agree your goals in a work setting, and fully buy into them when they are personal, and not take on anything that sets you up for unnecessary failure.

Of course, we all set goals for ourselves whether we realise it or not, because the majority of things that we want to happen in the future are essentially goals. But thinking vaguely about what we want further down the road is much less effective than actively forging and refining our goals as we move through life. This is something that really hit home with me after my diagnosis because I wanted to find a way to feel more in control of my destiny, even though there was a limit to what I could do in the face of cancer. Setting goals was by definition a positive thing to do, as it involved taking control of the direction I was travelling in. Rather than letting the chips fall where they may or blindly accepting my fate, I reclaimed agency and acted to overcome the problems I was facing. But saying I wanted to live wasn't specific enough – I needed to come up with achievable goals that would help me to live a healthy and happy life for as long as possible.

So what does it take to turn an idea for something we'd like to achieve in the future into a capital-G Goal like wanting to live? And how do we know that the goals we have are moving us in the right direction? As a means of judging whether your goals are the right ones or whether it might be time to set some new ones, have a think about your life right now and what you most want to change. It doesn't have to be something colossal, a seismic life shift, and it doesn't have to be a complete 180-degree about turn from where you are right now. Whatever means something to you is important; it doesn't matter if it's not going to change the world. Maybe you want to alter the way you operate at work or in your relationship. Maybe you don't feel your voice is loud enough and you want to change that. Maybe you're always apologising for yourself and don't want to any more. Maybe you want to feel fitter before Christmas, eat more fruit and vegetables and less red meat, or drink less alcohol during the week. Once you've done this, write down a list of your goals, big and small, that relate to what it is that you most want in life right now. As you are doing so, think about these three key questions:

1. How important is the goal to you?
2. How confident are you about accomplishing the goal?
3. How consistent is the goal with your values and beliefs?

The goals you decide to include on your list once you've thought about these questions can be big things you need to build up to step by step or they can be micro goals, and you need both in your life. Small goals for me have been things like getting through my next chemo cycle without a panic attack or drinking a green smoothie every day. My micro goals have all contributed to the macro one – living. What are your micro goals and what are the big goals that they are taking you towards?

Another useful way to check that the goals you have written down are the right ones is to apply the 'three Es'. Your goals should:

1. **Enlighten**: reveal your strengths and weaknesses, show you what you want to achieve and help you to prioritise.
2. **Encourage**: provide you with motivation, boost your confidence and give you courage to execute your plans.
3. **Enable**: help you to build skills, enhance your efficiency and assist you in implementing your plans.

In the past, you might have heard other people suggest that you should write down your goals if you want to make them happen. Those people often reference a well-known study in psychology, sometimes said to have taken place at Harvard and sometimes at Yale, into the positive effect of writing down your goals. It found that the 3 per cent of undergraduates who made a list of goals for their future were found to be earning a staggering ten times more than the rest of their fellow students twenty years later. The only problem with this study is that it never took place.

Once it was revealed that this often-quoted study was a myth, researcher Gail Matthews decided to explore whether there was actually any truth in the idea that writing down your goals is beneficial. She set up a study in which she divided the participants into five groups, each of which was asked to do one more thing to commit to their goals than the last group. The first was simply asked to think about what they wanted to achieve over the next four weeks. The second was asked to do the same but had to write their goals down. The third group also had to come up with concrete ways in which they would make their goals happen, which Matthews called 'action commitments', the fourth shared their written goals and action commitments with a supportive friend and, finally, the fifth group had to do all of this but also send weekly progress reports to their supportive friend.

The findings were clear: the more specific and actionable the goals were, and the more committed and account-able the participants were, the more they achieved over the four-week period. In fact, each group achieved more than the previous one, demonstrating that it is definitely worth making a list of your goals, but only if you follow the blueprint of group five and reinforce your intentions with actions that will help to make things happen.

Another great way of making sure you can accomplish your goals is to check them using SMART criteria, which is something you may well have come across before, especially in a work setting. It's a tool that originally came out of management theory, and I know it might sound really boring, but it's actually applicable to lots of things, and I've used it throughout my life, before and after cancer. The idea is that it helps you to refine what it is you really want and focus your energies so you can get there. Think about something you'd love to do in the near future and see how it measures up to the five categories below:

1. **Specific**: if your goal is too vague, it makes it more difficult to put in place the steps to reach it. Instead of saying, 'I want to be successful,' it is better to say what you want to be successful at.

2. **Measurable**: you need to be able to tell if you have reached your goal, as well as being able to monitor your progress along the way. So what will a successful outcome actually look like?

3. **Achievable**: the more challenging your goal, the more you can get out of it, but it can't be so difficult

as to make it impossible. How demoralising would that be! I'm not going to break the marathon world record, so there's no point making that one of my goals.

4. **Realistic**: related to achievability, a goal also needs to be constrained by reality. In other words, it needs to be within your power to make it happen, and it helps if it plays to your strengths. If there is no way of making the time in your life right now to commit to the project to get it to where you want it to be, then maybe you need to reassess.

5. **Timely**: this can mean that the time is right for that particular goal, or it can refer to the time frame in which the goal should be achieved.

Here's what happens when I apply SMART to my primary goal – to live:

Specific: very! Keep on breathing, keep putting one foot in front of the other and keep getting back up again when it all gets too much.

Measurable: my days, weeks and months mark the passage of time during which I achieve my goal. I have work projects I meet, deadlines I work to, podcasts and interviews I record. And my health at any given time is something that can be monitored and quantified.

Achievable: yes, for now, but whether it'll stay that way is out of my hands.

Realistic: yes and no. In the face of an incurable diagnosis, you could argue it's not, but there are things I can do to increase my chances, like exercising, eating well and participating fully in my treatment.

Timely: yes, it's what I need right now.

If I've convinced you to make a proper list of your goals, take a few minutes to look them over and ask yourself whether they are SMART using the criteria above. For example, if your aim is to learn a new language, can you carve out enough hours in your week to make it achievable? Is wanting to 'get fit' specific enough? Do you have an event you're working towards taking part in, a distance to run, a time to aim for? Setting an achievable *and* aspirational target is a skill in itself. And asking yourself how you know if you've set the right goal is one of the hardest parts. If you want to qualify for the Boston Marathon, but your time is 13 minutes off what you need to qualify, should you stick with that goal and feel like a failure if you don't hit the mark or should you find a more realistic, achievable goal? That's not an easy question to answer, so perhaps you could start by breaking the problem down into smaller parts: how much training have you been doing? How much progress have you made so far? How much time have you got? Do you have the capacity to train more and therefore improve enough to meet the qualifying mark in the time available? And do you actually still want to do this? When you sit down and imagine running the Boston Marathon, does it make you feel happy and fulfilled enough that the commitment to extra training feels worth it, or does it just make you feel tired and under pressure? (If so, perhaps your time is a reflection of the fact that you're doing less training than you meant to because you're really not enjoying it.) If after doing this work you conclude that the goal is achievable and you still want to do it, even if it is going to be difficult, it is worth pursuing.

Once you've set or recalibrated your goals and you're (hopefully!) feeling excited and motivated to get started, try not to overdo it to begin with. If you set yourself too many goals, you can easily become overwhelmed and give up before you've even got started. A few to begin with is fine. If setting more concrete goals in the way I've described is new to you, it probably also makes sense to focus on short-term goals at first – once you start to achieve these and benefit from the feeling that frequent success brings, the more ready you will be to take on more goals, including longer-term ones. Finally, try to frame your goals as positively as you can. Instead of saying that you want to lose weight, decide that you want to eat more healthily and exercise more. Goals should feel like something positive that you are excited to work towards – not a punishment and not something you are doing because someone else has made you feel like you should.

Goals should feel like something positive that you are excited to work towards.

* * *

Only 20 per cent of people carry their New Year's resolutions into February. Why? Because when it comes to these types of resolutions, we often set ourselves up for failure. When was the last time your New Year's resolution was something achievable? Millions of people across the UK wake up on 1 January and resolve to reduce their alcohol intake. But what does 'reduce' actually mean, and what steps are they going to take to make it happen?

When you set yourself a goal, no amount of wishing will make it a reality. Unless you take steps to set yourself up for success, you'll fail. In the classroom, good teachers don't allow their students to keep doing the same thing over and over again, failing each time. We encourage them to take more time, ask a friend, review what they've done to see what they got wrong – in other words, we get them to implement lots of micro steps to set them up for success.

I've seen so many times that young people find it easier to believe in themselves when someone else believes in them, and we know as adults that self-belief is a huge driver of success. But as adults, none of us have a teacher who'll tell us we're predicted an A grade, so we have to become that voice for ourselves. We have to believe in ourselves and set expectations high enough to be worthwhile, but realistic enough so they're achievable.

So don't then rest on your laurels. Don't be the person who waits and researches rather than takes active steps towards what they want. Don't assume you have all the time in the world, because you might not. Get urgent and get moving. A plan to reach your goal is only useful if you execute it. And don't just look at your goals as things you want to get to at some point. If they are important enough to you, they are worth making a part of your everyday life. How are you going to get there? What steps will you be taking along the way? How are you going to make the time to dedicate to them? Start today with urgency and set yourself up to win. That's what I've tried to do, especially when things have been at their most difficult. It would have been easy to stop planning for the future when I found out my cancer was incurable, but continuing to assess my goals and set new ones has given me purpose and something to strive for, whether that was my blog in the early days or my newspaper column and media appearances as I worked to get the message out about bowel cancer. And this, in turn, has kept me engaged in the business of living a good life, one full of interest and love and happiness.

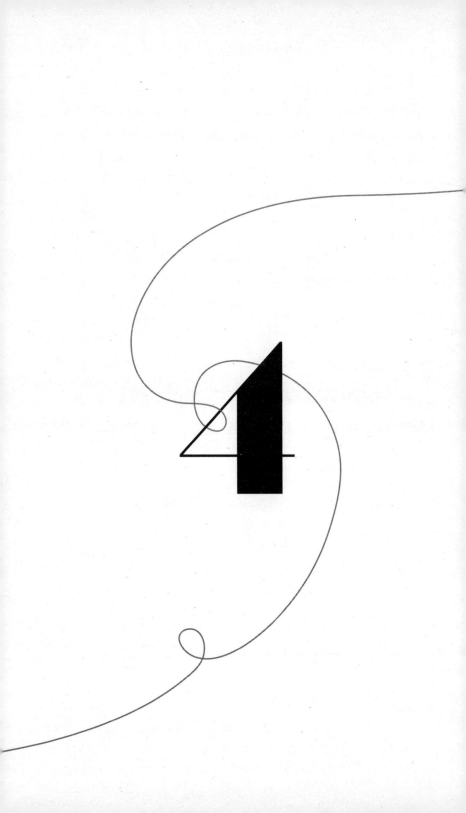

how I've kept **going**
when I felt like stopping

'The most efficient way to live reasonably is every morning to make a plan of one's day and every night to examine the results obtained'

Alexis Carrel

During my years as a teacher, I worked according to an hour-by-hour timetable, in which the structure of my day was dictated to me. Teaching is one of those jobs where you don't have the option to change things around or just not show up. You can't move a class because you don't feel like it or because something's overrun. You have to be there, because if you don't turn up, or even if you do but you haven't planned your lesson, 30 kids will soon create absolute chaos. Teaching felt like a huge responsibility to me, but I really loved it, and it also defined the structure of my life.

When I was in the classroom and working towards becoming a head teacher, milestones were marked out for me; terms and school holidays gave my life a predictable shape, and the annual exam results told me how well I was doing and gave me the opportunity to pause, reflect and move forward meaningfully, always striving to do better. Exam results were very public markers – some excited parents would write to tell me how delighted they were with their children's grades, while others would be upset that their children unfortunately had to do resits. When that was all taken away from me, it felt like a huge blow and I had to re-evaluate so many things.

When I was diagnosed with cancer and it became clear that I couldn't work any more, I no longer had a routine that made me get up in the morning. For ages, all I could see was my failure at living and a vast expanse where my career had once been. And that was quite a struggle – the fact is, if I don't have something to get up for, I don't get up. Before cancer, I was quite hard-nosed about getting on with things, even if I was ill. Like a lot of people who are dedicated to their careers, I didn't feel as though I had the option to say, 'I'm having a bad day. I can't go in.'

So it probably comes as no surprise that one of my main coping mechanisms following my cancer diagnosis has been to keep really busy. Finding a new routine to help me achieve the goals I set for myself (as we discussed in the previous chapter) was so important in getting me back on my feet after my diagnosis, and I think it is a strategy that can help other people in times of adversity, although I appreciate it might not be the best approach, or even possible, for everybody. It can be as simple as starting with putting one thing a day in your schedule, even if that's just saying, 'I am going to go for a walk this afternoon.' I have found that it's also beneficial if you plan something at the same time every day. There's a reason that if you see a therapist, they make you commit to a certain time each week, and it's because structure is part of the change they want to help you bring about in your life.

When I am well enough, my daily routine is very straightforward. I'm definitely not a morning person, but I make

Finding a new routine was so important in getting me back on my feet.

myself get up and do some exercise followed by some breakfast. And I don't always know what is going to happen after that, but those three things are the cornerstone of the new structure that I've had to build. It probably doesn't sound like a lot, but it gives my day focus and helps me to get going, and sometimes that's all you need to start the day in a positive way. I know it's really helped me to pick myself up again. Of course, some people find routine more challenging, and it can be hard to stick to one, but it can be extremely beneficial as a first step in overcoming the challenges that you face.

I also recognise that it is difficult to introduce routine into your life if you don't have any external forces prompting you to do something. If I have a weekend without any other commitments, it's not unheard of for me to get out of bed at about midday and move to the sofa and not leave until it is time to go to bed again! And while sometimes I do need to recharge my batteries, most of the time I have to recognise that doing nothing like this only makes me feel crap about myself, because I feel as though I am going backwards and not making any progress.

Of course, if what you really need is a rest, and forcing yourself through the motions of your routine will only make you feel worse, then you need to listen to that. It's interesting – if I say on social media that I've gone for a walk, I get loads of people congratulating me for getting moving and equally loads of people telling me to take it easy! I have come to realise that often it's a case of people projecting their own situations on to me. Not everyone wants to hear all about what someone else has achieved if they are struggling. It's about focusing on yourself and doing what is right for you at any given moment.

The reality for me is that I need to have at least one little thing to aim for each day. And it needs to be something achievable (I told you those SMART criteria would come in handy). It might be that I've taken the dog for a walk. It might be that I've cooked one meal. Whatever it is, it gives my day the little bit of structure that I need. I have a friend with a nine-year-old daughter called Annie who is a big fan of making lists. The very first thing she puts on a list is always 'make a list' – that way, by the time she's finished writing it, she can already tick off the top task! It's a simple example, but it sets her up for success and makes her feel positive.

If I'm going through a bad patch and wake up in the morning feeling like I can't get going, I will plan my day down to 15- to 30-minute slots:

- 9am: brush my teeth and wash my hair
- 9.15am: eat breakfast
- 9.45am: check my emails
- 10am: look on social media for 15 minutes
- 10.15am: have a cup of tea
- 10.30am: record an ad for a brand I'm working with

It can be as basic as this, but it's a guideline to follow when I don't know how to get through my day. I use the notes app on my phone, and I have days and days and days of these types of schedules, probably coinciding with some of my darkest moments. For somebody else, it might look totally different. Or you might be thinking, 'God, I can't function like that!'

I need to have at least one little thing to aim for each day.

If I'm in a more normal headspace, I instead create to-do lists with just the main things that I want to get done by the end of the day – email this person, do this meeting – and I don't feel I need to include things like 'get dressed'. However, if I'm in a bad headspace, I break things down into manageable chunks and always include things that I know I can do, such as clean my teeth, because it feels really good when you can tick them off.

Anyone who's followed me for a while knows that the summer is my favourite time of the year, and my aim now is to try to fit in a few events while I'm still here and able to. But be under no illusion, I've worked out that it takes me longer to get ready and organised to go than the time I actually last anywhere. Getting dressed is exhausting, getting my meds organised is a faff, the extra moving, the travel, the wondering what mood your stomach is in – it's all real. But then the feeling of making it to something you didn't think possible – like my visits to Glyndebourne opera house and Royal Ascot in June 2022 – having put on make-up, donned new shoes, with the sunshine smiling down – well, then it's all worth it. And making to-do lists to get me there, even if they're now only in my head, is a kind of cheeky 'still living while dying' two fingers up to it all.

People often say to me, 'How do you get through a day?' But sometimes you don't have to get through the day. You just have to get through the next hour, the next minute, the next few seconds. I get that this prescriptive approach doesn't work for everybody, but it really works for me and is a strategy that allows me to carry on.

Scheduling my time gives me a sense of achievement in two ways: first, I am more organised, use my days effectively and don't forget things because my goals and commitments are written down. I don't end the day and suddenly remember something that I wanted to do, that I had the time and energy to accomplish but just forgot about. Second, just like Annie, I also get to tick things off once I've completed them, which gives me a sense of achievement. Never underestimate the jolt of positivity you get from ticking something off a list!

People often say the reason they have failed at something is because of time: 'I didn't have time to train properly'; 'I didn't have enough time to revise'. Scheduling your time properly and making to-do lists of what you need to achieve in that period, whether that be a day, a week, a month or a year, reduces the likelihood that time will be the reason for you not completing what you want to get done – just ask the GCSE student who writes up a revision timetable and sticks to it meticulously.

If you're a high achiever with lots on your plate, your list might contain things like 'finalise the big deal'. If you're in the grip of anxiety or another mental health condition, your list might have 'wash my hair' and 'make my bed' on it. It doesn't matter what's on your list. What matters is that it works for you. When you plan and structure, the chances of failure are reduced because less is left to chance, and if you do happen to fail, you can use it as an opportunity to learn and have another go (which I go into in more detail in Chapter 5).

* * *

As I said in the last chapter, my goal is to live, but it's also to live well, and that means taking care of myself, eating right, exercising, making time for the people I love and creating quality connections. Each time I accomplish one of those things, I pause, reflect and am thankful. Many of us will have used the idea of 'milestones' in our work lives as a means of monitoring our progress, and research has shown that, when it comes to work, teams presented with frequent milestones outperform those that aren't. There are also certain things in our personal lives that we usually mark as milestones, such as birthdays and anniversaries. That said, a staggering 46 per cent of Brits don't even bother celebrating their wedding anniversary. That's almost half of all couples in the UK who think it's a milestone that doesn't have to be marked, despite a wedding day being one of the most important days in anyone's life!

Milestones are a way of putting down markers in your life and judging how far you have travelled towards achieving the goals that we discussed in the previous chapter. They don't always have to be about celebrating success – they can be about acknowledging another step away from trauma or something that's been holding you back. That's what people who attend support groups such as Alcoholics Anonymous do – they celebrate the days since their last drink. At their core, milestones are about reflecting on your progress, and they also break long projects into manageable chunks. They present us with an opportunity to take stock, look at how far we've come, assess what we've learned, analyse what went right and wrong, and congratulate ourselves on our efforts so far before we keep moving forward. They're a much-needed pit stop that can help us gather energy and momentum to keep going and get ourselves ever closer to the finish line. But what if we started to apply those 'stopping to take a breath' moments more frequently? Rather than just marking the occasions that are expected of us, what if we paused and smelled the roses a bit more? What if we congratulated ourselves on the small things – those less common milestones that we can all find and celebrate – and stopped and looked at how far we'd come?

Milestones are a way of judging how far you have travelled towards achieving your goals.

If being told that you only have an 8 per cent chance of living for five years is not a mortal line in the sand, then I don't know what is. On 16 December every year – the day I received my incurable diagnosis – I acknowledge the milestone of another year living with this terrible illness. It's not one that elicits unbridled joy, but that's OK. Milestones don't have to be something you break out the bubbly and balloons for – they can be a reminder of trauma too and how far you've come to cope with or move past it.

When I got to my first year, though, there was cause to celebrate. I'd defied the odds and was still alive. Years two and three were quite scary, because most people with my condition die at that point. Year four was a weird feeling because I really acknowledged that to get to this point was huge from a statistical point of view. Year five was an even more momentous occasion – 92 people out of 100 don't get this opportunity and I did. I made it to my fortieth birthday and the five-year mark, and, on 16 December 2016, I never thought I would do either of those things.

It is a similar situation with my treatment. When you're told you have to have X number of chemotherapy treatments or X number of radiotherapy sessions, you count them off. I certainly did at the start. But I'm a long-term cancer patient now – and there are a few of us at the Royal Marsden, where I received my treatment. One is called John, and he's had cancer for 30 years. He was diagnosed in the 1990s, and he's lived with cancer ever since. It's metastasised since his initial testicular cancer diagnosis, and he's in his sixties now. Then there's Marjorie, who has had cancer for 20 years. We're like a little club, but I've only just been admitted. When I was first diagnosed, they whipped me under their wing, and since then I've seen them do the same with so many other patients who come through the door petrified of what lies ahead.

When anyone with cancer starts their journey, there are the milestones you can't help but observe: first and last chemo sessions, or the number of radiotherapy sessions to go. But when you're a long-term cancer patient like John and Marjorie, what do you do then? When I last caught up with John, he told me he'd now had 252 cycles of chemotherapy. It had become a bit of a comical milestone to him, but it was still a milestone and deserved to be observed – in his case with a bit of a laugh.

I think that if you celebrate the milestones on your journey, you'll program your brain to desire more success. If your goal is to run a 5k in less than 30 minutes, you should be fist-pumping-whooping-and-hollering happy for any PB you make that gets you closer to that mark. Rewarding the parts of a journey instead of just the destination makes you want more of the behaviour that caused the success – in other words, the hard work.

Taking stock of the steps towards our goals improves our chances of success as well as sustaining and invigorating us along the way. Have you heard of the concept of 'chunking'? It isn't a very sexy word, I'll grant you, but it's exactly what I want you to think about. If you break down your larger goals into smaller chunks, then you can look at completing each one as moving you incrementally forward and as a milestone on the way to success. The journey is as vital as the destination, so make sure it's a path you're happy to be on and enjoy the incremental successes and celebrate the small, hard-fought wins as well as the big, shiny achievements.

* * *

What will success mean for you on your own personal journey? Success is different for everyone, and ideally it should be something we define ourselves and value for what it means to us, and not because of how we think other people perceive our achievements. For me, success is living and defying the odds – but it's also managing to run a sub-30-minute 5k and decluttering my wardrobe.

Success can be something external that is visible to others or it can be something internal. Both are valid, but I would argue that seeking acknowledgement for your successes isn't always healthy. Is the sense of reinforcement you get from congratulations on social media posts something you really need to feel like you're succeeding? If you're reading this having checked your social media in the last few hours for likes or retweets, you're not alone! It's hard to resist. The thing is, though, true self-worth comes from within, not from how many people like your latest post or follow you on Twitter or Instagram. It might sound a bit trite, but others won't value you until you can learn to value yourself.

One hurdle I can't get over – but I'm constantly trying to – is how badly I want acknowledgement for my successes. I used to be rewarded for my achievements all the time when I was a teacher, in terms of both the progress of my students and my own career advancement, and I'm still programmed to want that validation now – I know I don't need it any more, but that doesn't help the teacher in me who wants other people to know that I'm still moving forward.

When someone takes steps to improve their health, starts training for a marathon or goes vegan, other people often give positive reinforcement for those behaviours. But there aren't any congratulations for self-growth. No one cares that I'm healing or growing because they can't see it and it doesn't directly affect them.

When you're deciding on your goals and what it will mean to achieve them, think about what success really looks like – to you. I'm living every day as well as I can. I'm a successful author, podcast presenter, campaigner and columnist, and those things get me a lot of external praise and acknowledgement, but one of the things I'm most proud of is the difference I make to the dying and the bereaved.

A while ago, I received a message on social media from a bereft husband. His wife had died at home from bowel cancer just 30 minutes before he messaged me. In his sea of grief, he reached out to me and thanked me for my podcast *You, Me and the Big C*. He told me his wife had avidly followed me and that I'd given her hope and reassurance, particularly in the final moments of her life. He thanked me for keeping her going while cancer had ravaged her body.

Then, a few weeks ago, I received a message from a woman who was holding her mother's hand as she was dying from cancer in a hospice. The daughter had been told her mother wouldn't live through the night, and yet in her maelstrom of grief she'd reached out to me to thank me for the podcast they'd listened to together.

Neither of those examples are what people might traditionally refer to as successes. They were private messages in the midst of grief and cancer and death. As an ex-teacher who likes visible metrics of progress, I didn't think of them as successes at first – they felt raw and emotional and incredibly sad. But looking at them in retrospect and through a different prism, I've come to realise that I've had a huge amount of success in sharing my story and giving a little bit of comfort to people going through the same thing as me. How fortunate am I that in the midst of that level of trauma people feel they can get in touch with me about how they're feeling? It's a very positive side effect of being a podcast presenter and author, and not one I ever even thought about when I first started. It just goes to show that success comes in many different forms, and it's not necessarily about rewards or acknowledgement or praise.

It's often the intangible things that mean the most when you take time to recognise them. It's not always about marking the big, earth-shattering events or achievements – the incremental successes that bring a smile or a sense of relief are just as important, as is the positivity that you put out into the world and the difference you can make to others. Maybe you aced a day of homeschooling when the country was locked down during the Covid-19 pandemic – you might not have thought of it as a big life achievement or something to be really proud of, but helping your child to thrive in such extraordinary circumstances is absolutely a success, and you should stop and take stock of it. If you think back on the last 24 hours, I'll bet that there are plenty of small successes you ignored when they happened – maybe it was checking in on a relative or neighbour, making the kids a lunch they devoured, putting clean bed sheets on or going for a walk in the park that you enjoyed. The banner moments in life will always give you the most satisfaction, but the steps along the way are what make the journey enjoyable – that's where the living really happens; something I've come to appreciate more and more over the last five years.

In teaching, you're trained to praise the effort more than the outcome, and we need to apply that to our own lives, observing milestones as we go. I mark milestones in my struggle with cancer because I shouldn't really be here, but they're not the only milestones that are important to me. Parenting successes, phoning a friend I haven't been in touch with for a while

Success comes in many different forms.

or helping someone I haven't even met are also worth celebrating and what keep me going day to day. If you're working hard towards a life goal, it's vital you take time every now and then to pat yourself on the back and take stock of all the things you have already succeeded at – the things you have in the here and now. The path to success is paved with small wins if you only take the time to notice them.

'The key to realizing a dream
is to focus not on success but
significance, and then even the
small steps and little victories
along your path will take
on greater meaning'

Oprah Winfrey

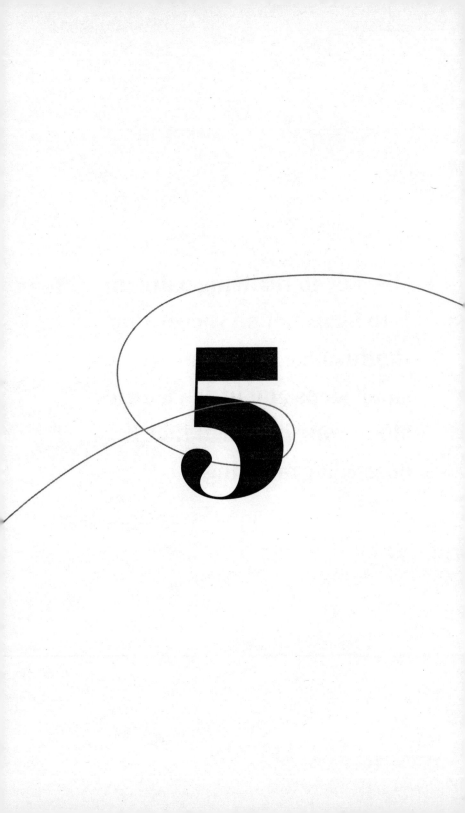

fuel the fire
of failure

'It is impossible to live without failing at something, unless you live so cautiously that you might as well not have lived at all – in which case you fail by default'

J. K. Rowling

Right now, I'm failing big time. I'm failing to live. And it's not my fault. My body doesn't work – I have little control over my cancer and, honestly, that sucks.

Of course, having cancer isn't really a 'failing' and it's not something I can fix, but what no one told me at the time of my diagnosis, and what I have had to teach myself, is that while my odds of still being here in the foreseeable future might not look great, I do have a 100 per cent chance to get smarter every day that I live. I've realised that I have to find ways to feel as though I'm winning even though my life will be cut short. Even the failure of my body is an opportunity to learn something and to grow. So, while I'm still here, I'm learning and living every single day, keeping myself busy and trying, failing and learning constantly.

Seeing the benefits of failure is not something that necessarily comes easily, though, particularly not as we reach adulthood. It's a different story when we're young. One of the best things about watching an infant learn to do something new is how they're not scared of failure – they'll fall and get straight back up again. When they first try to use a spoon, they'll keep smearing whatever it is they are supposed to be eating all over their faces until they get the hang of it with absolutely no embarrassment whatsoever. But at some point, self-awareness kicks in and kids stop instinctively understanding failure as a part of learning and start to worry about how they'll be perceived by adults and their peers when they get things wrong.

By the time they reach secondary school, failure is seen as 'losing'. I think social media has a part to play in this – and not just for young people – because it shows us successes the majority of the time. We see curated images, a showreel of the best bits. We are shown a beautiful cake, but not the first attempt that fell apart and went in the bin. We'll post a picture of the gorgeous cottage we're staying in, but not the motorway we didn't know was at the end of the garden when we booked it. That's understandable – the world doesn't necessarily want to see pictures of these things! But if we constantly celebrate 'perfection' and never see the things that don't go right, we're potentially encouraging children – and adults – to veer away from things they might fail at. We come to believe that failure is something to avoid at all costs, rather than the incredible learning tool that it is. And that perspective may unfortunately stay with many of us throughout our lives. It's one of the main reasons that I've tried to be as frank about

While I'm still here, I'm learning and living every single day.

the realities of my situation on social media, on my podcast and in my writing – I want people to understand what it's really like to have cancer, warts and all.

Teachers build failure into their lessons. For example, if you're brand new to the concept of algebra, your teacher will expect it to take you a while to get the hang of it, so they'll factor failure time into the lesson. Educators see students' first attempts at anything as just that – attempts. Subsequent attempts will see fewer and fewer failures as knowledge and experience build – in other words, those first failures are both inevitable and vital to ensuring ultimate success.

But, as adults, how often do we give ourselves time to fail and factor in a few goes before we get it right? None of us knows everything, yet we think we should be able to succeed more than we realistically can. We tend to focus on failure as a lack of success, of falling short and not being good enough. But when you see failure as an invitation to try again, as an opportunity to have another swing of the bat, you begin to turn that definition on its head. All the time I spent in the classroom, watching kids get it wrong and then eventually get it right, showed me that with a positive mindset we can learn some very important lessons from failure and embrace the opportunity to have another go, this time armed with all the information that failure gave us.

How we perceive failures, both in the instant they happen and in retrospect, very much determines how much we can take from them. We have to be willing to look for the lessons failure is trying to teach us rather than wallowing in disappointment. I believe that failing is brilliant; it's one of the best life lessons we can ever get – we just have to be open to the learning opportunities it offers, rather than get bogged down by the negative associations of the word itself.

We have to be willing to look for the lessons failure is trying to teach us.

If you've never failed, it might mean you've never really pushed yourself all that hard, because, in my opinion, it's impossible to thrive and live life to the fullest without failure. Not only is there more satisfaction in achieving something difficult after trying a number of times, but failure is also a tool that we can harness if we have the right mindset.

* * *

It's one thing to say that failure is an invaluable way to learn and change, but of course it's not always easy to put that philosophy into practice day to day, through the dark moments when I am in pain and faced with thoughts of all the things I won't get to experience in the future. One thing that has really helped me is my background as a teacher and all I learned through my professional life about the importance of growth and the power of the mind.

Before my cancer diagnosis, I already believed that attitude and mindset are hugely important to how you process and react to what life throws at you and go a long way towards predicting whether you stagnate or thrive. My experiences of the last five years have absolutely confirmed this for me. A shitty situation is a shitty situation, but your mindset is what affects how you feel about it, what you do about it and, in most cases, the outcome. Most importantly, having a positive mindset can help you to navigate life's unexpected shocks and learn from when things go wrong, as they inevitably do.

There are lots of theories about mindset, but the one that I first came across, and that really made me think, was the idea of fixed and growth mindsets, as defined by the eminent psychologist Carol Dweck. If you've ever done any leadership training or read business books – or, indeed, you work in education – you will probably have heard of this. Dweck explains that a fixed mindset is when you believe that creativity, intelligence and character are static and can't be changed. So if you're bad at maths, art or music it's because you just don't have those skills, or if you're brilliant at sport, writing and dance then that's because you were born with an innate talent for them. A fixed mindset, in its most simplistic form, is one whereby we believe that we're pretty much set from day one, as a result of our genes, in what we can and can't do, and what we're good and bad at. In certain situations, having a fixed mindset could be a good thing. Some entrepreneurs, for example, could be said to have fixed mindsets. They veer away from things they perceive themselves to be bad at, avoiding situations where they believe they might fail, thus making success more likely. For the most part, however, a fixed mindset has been shown to limit success.

A growth mindset is essentially the opposite. It's generally defined as a belief that creativity, intelligence and character are flexible and can be changed by hard work, dedication and effort. That nothing is set in stone. That you can evolve and grow and achieve – with the right mindset.

Dweck became interested in mindset when she observed that people deal with failure in very different ways. Some people, when faced with a difficult problem or a setback, give up, whereas others see adversity as a challenge and are spurred on by it. These latter people don't just seem to cope with failure; they appear to welcome it and thrive on it. It became apparent to Dweck that these people did not believe they weren't clever or skilled enough to overcome the obstacles they faced – they believed they could improve and that failure is, in fact, how you learn.

Dweck argues it's 'not ability or belief in that ability that predicts resilience and perseverance in the face of challenge and failure', it is the 'individual's belief about the nature of ability'. It's not about being successful or achieving in isolation; it's about believing you can learn when things go wrong as much as you can learn when they go right. You need to trust the fact you can develop and grow – you have to see abilities as fluid and able to increase and flourish through hard work, grit and resilience. Having that frame of mind has allowed me to adapt to the realities of my life with cancer, revealing qualities I didn't know I had and turning what I perceived to be weaknesses into strengths.

'When you change the way you look at things, the things you look at change'

Dr Wayne Dyer

It's also worth considering that our emotions, expectations and preconceived ideas have a big impact on what we even consider as 'failure'. It might seem like it's binary – you either got it right or wrong, got the job or didn't, hit your training target or fell short – but one person's failure is another person's change of direction. Consider, too, that when we move on from a 'failure' and it fades into the past, how we view it can change.

Author Susan Cain once described herself as an 'ambivalent corporate attorney'. She didn't love her work, but she did it well and was on track for a partnership in her law firm . . . until one day she was told she wouldn't be put up for partner. She broke down, asked for a leave of absence and then remembered she wanted to be a writer. That same day, she started writing. She eventually wrote the bestseller *Quiet*, an expertly researched and highly engaging book that's inspired countless introverts to find their place in the world.

Although Susan failed to gain a partnership, she was able to reframe the situation as an opportunity and learn something in the process: that she was pursuing a career she didn't care about instead of following her dream to be a writer. This insight wasn't necessarily immediate – that fateful day, she might have considered it a failure. Today, I'm sure she'd call it one of the best things that ever happened to her. And I'm equally sure there are things in all of our lives that at one time seemed like failures but, with hindsight, we have come to realise taught us something important.

Think about the path your failures have put you on and what you've garnered from the journey. Even if your failure landed you at rock bottom and you can't see any positive in it right now, that's OK, because you now only have one way to go and that's up.

You can evolve and grow and achieve – with the right mindset.

A lot of the critical thinking about what failure is comes from business. Amy Edmondson, a professor at Harvard Business School, says there are three main types of failure:

1. Avoidable or preventable
2. Unavoidable or complex
3. Fast or intellectual

Some are more useful than others, but all have something to teach us. Learning from mistakes isn't always easy, and many of us resort to the blame game when things go wrong. That is why correctly identifying which category a failure falls into is so useful.

Lots of times, when things don't go to plan, there is a very good reason why not. Maybe you didn't dot every 'i' or cross every 't'. Perhaps you miscalculated the importance of something or you didn't ask for help when it was needed. These are **avoidable failures** where the outcome might have been better had you done things differently. You can't always see ahead of time what might be an avoidable failure because they often only present themselves in hindsight, but sometimes you'll kick yourself because you might have been able to see them coming with enough forethought. By assessing in retrospect what went wrong and why, you can better position yourself to avoid making the same mistakes in the future and thereby increase your chances of success.

A case in point: my sister-in-law Clare Bowen set up the Royal Parks Half Marathon in 2008 and, in the years before my diagnosis, I had taken part every year. But in 2017, after finding out I had cancer, I decided I would sit it out. When my amazing friends heard this, they said that they would run on my behalf, which I thought was such a wonderful gesture. However, when the day arrived, I got really upset – it was heartbreaking to stand by and watch when all I wanted was to be out there with them. I vowed that the following year I would run again – I wasn't going to let cancer stop me.

I signed up for the 2018 run, but I didn't tell anyone I was participating. I was still pretty fit at that point, as I have always tried to blend exercise with my illness, and I figured I could just decide on the day if I was up for it. I had run 10k on numerous occasions, and I thought

I could always just walk the remaining kilometres if I ran out of steam at any point.

A few days before the event, my good friend Rachael Bland died, and I thought, 'Screw this, I'm going to get a T-shirt with her face on it and do the run in her memory.' I hadn't really prepared for a half marathon, and I hadn't run that distance in quite some time, but I thought I could wing it.

On the day, I ran with Clare and it started off well. I was filled with adrenalin, and this carried me for the first few kilometres. It wasn't long, though, before I started to feel some pain in my ankle. The buzz of the day and the pride I felt at being there meant I kept going. Eventually, the pain got too much to run, so we walked the remainder of the way. As soon as we finished and the adrenalin left my body, I realised my ankle was seriously hurt. We visited the event medics, who quickly whisked me off to A&E, where they discovered I had a stress fracture. I ended up in a big ugly boot for weeks – I even had to attend some fancy award ceremonies wearing it alongside my glamorous dresses!

Looking back, this was completely avoidable. I didn't prepare properly before doing the run, and I didn't listen to my body when it was telling me there was something wrong. It took me six months to get back to running again, but I learned from this failure and didn't make the same mistake again. When I went a step further and ran the London Marathon in 2020, I was ready for it thanks to the lessons learned from this entirely preventable failure.

Sometimes in life, though, no matter how well you have prepared, things still go wrong because of complex factors that couldn't have been predicted. It is tempting in such instances to say that nothing can be learned from these **unavoidable failures**. I disagree. It is still valuable to look back and work out why things went wrong, as, armed with this new information, perhaps you can turn an unavoidable failure into an avoidable one next time. But there is also a lesson to be learned just from the fact of failing – that life doesn't always run smoothly and some things are out of your control: a cancer diagnosis, your car being rear-ended, a global pandemic. These are bolt-from-the-blue acts that upend even the best-laid plans and are completely out of our hands, so we can't allow ourselves to be too disheartened by them.

There was nothing I could do to avoid getting cancer, and there is nothing I can do to change it now. It is easy to look for someone or something to blame in situations such as this, and I definitely went through that process when I was first diagnosed. Despite being a healthy vege-tarian, doing regular exercise and being younger than the average bowel-cancer patient, I spent quite a long time blaming myself for not going to the GP, saying to myself,

I should have done this, I should have done that; I should have pushed more.

I knew something wasn't right with my body, and I kept going for check-ups, but my symptoms were dismissed as being caused by anxiety or irritable bowel syndrome. That, sadly, wasn't the case. But, at the end of the day, nothing I could have done would have changed the outcome for me. It couldn't be avoided, and I eventually realised that trying to attribute blame was pointless. Instead, I decided to do something useful and campaign to raise awareness of the disease and its symptoms. The most important thing is how you respond to an unavoidable failure.

'Do not wait; the time will never be "just right". Start where you stand, and work with whatever tools you may have at your command, and better tools will be found as you go along'

Napoleon Hill

Popular in business, **fast failures**, which I like to think of as 'give-it-a-go' failures, are where you're keen to learn as much as you can as quickly as you can. You might also think of them as deliberate or iterative failures, as you expect that things will go wrong, but you decide to have a go anyway so that you can learn and improve. These are often low-level failures that we can learn from quickly, adapting and reapplying ourselves, before cracking on with the next attempt. They're unaware of it at the time, but toddlers learning to walk or feed themselves make these types of failures – they give things a go, and when they don't work out, they instantly try something different. These types of failures also occur when experimentation is required. Sometimes you just need to leap into the unknown and see what happens.

Between the ages of eight and fourteen, I was in the national gymnastics programme, and this kind of give-it-a-go failure was absolutely baked into the process. When attempting a new move, I couldn't simply do it first time; there was no expectation of success at the outset. Instead, I had to fail and get back up and rectify the problem or error. My coach had to teach me how, and I would also learn from others in the gym. It required a lot of support and building up to being able to perform the move. On the parallel bars, for example, I would start by falling into the cushioned pit beneath the apparatus without any expectation of catching the bar. I would then build up to having a teammate or coach underneath to catch me. Then, eventually, I might get to the point where I felt I could do it without so much padding beneath the bars and my coach standing by to help if need be. And I would have to repeat the move over and over again, learning from each failed attempt until I was confident with it and able to move on to the next thing.

Working through those attempts was so important. If you tried a new move without beginning at stage one, there was a very real possibility that you would break your neck. The reality is that you would never do that. I think sometimes we forget this and go straight in for the kill. Then, when we do fail, we do so catastrophically, because we haven't learned how to support ourselves along the way. Fast failures, on the other hand, acknowledge that you can't just skip to the end, and that sometimes you need to give things a go and see what happens. In this way, they allow for incremental improvement towards ultimate success.

> **'Ever tried. Ever failed. No matter. Try again. Fail again. Fail better'**
>
> **Samuel Beckett**

* * *

Fear of failure is something that holds us back and stops us from learning. But if we acknowledge that failure is an integral part of how we learn and grow, then it follows that it isn't something to shy away from or be ashamed of. So how do we best extract the lessons from failure? It's no good just saying that failure is OK because it is part of life and that we learn from our mistakes if we are not actively engaged in working out what those lessons are.

In teaching, one of the most important skills we try to develop in students is self-assessment. Children are taught to mark their own work, identify their mistakes (and what went well, of course) and begin to put things right. By doing so, they take on board the lessons from what went wrong much more effectively than when a teacher returns a marked piece of work covered in ticks and crosses, because children who are in control of their own learning and fully engaged in the process do better than those learning by rote.

In every single lesson I ever planned, I factored in some DIRT. That's 'Dedicated Improvement and Reflection Time' – the 'what can I learn' part of the lesson. DIRT is specifically allocated time for students to look at the work they've done to see where they've failed and assess how they could do it better. It's a sustainable cycle of self-reflection and taking on board feedback. But it's not just useful in the classroom – we all need to factor some DIRT into our lives.

Fear of failure is something that holds us back and stops us from learning.

Taking some time to look at what went wrong in order to arm you with the knowledge to help you get it right next time probably sounds pretty sensible and not that revolutionary. And yet how many of us are good at this kind of self-regulation? When we fail as adults, we often just try to forget about it and move on. The last time something went wrong, can you honestly say you analysed it and asked what went well, what could go better and what could be done differently next time? That's fantastic if you did, but, if not, I'd love you to consider doing so from now on. I promise that you'll cope with failure much better if you turn it into a self-regulating learning cycle.

Once you've decided to bring some DIRT into your life and reflect on the things that haven't gone as well as you hoped, the questions below might help you to get to the bottom of why not:

- What went wrong?
- What type of failure was it?
- What external factors had a bearing on it and what can you do to minimise their effect next time?
- Do you have what you need to fix the problem yourself or do you need to ask for help?
- How can you improve your chances of success in the future?
- What are the overall lessons learned?

There'll likely be many more questions you come up with yourself – the key is to focus on the details of what went wrong and what you can learn about yourself. Whenever you try something new or you set a goal for yourself, in addition to factoring in time to achieve what you set out to, if you include some DIRT in the process, you'll soon see the benefits.

Maybe you frequently start new exercise regimes but get bored and distracted and end up giving up. Maybe you always intend to eat healthily but get waylaid by the takeaway you walk past on the way home from work. Maybe your relationships have a tendency to play second fiddle to other aspects of your life. Whatever it is, DIRT will give you the space to identify the patterns of how and why things aren't working out for you. Once you've reflected on what went wrong, you can implement change, whether that's finding an exercise partner to help keep you motivated, walking a different way home or taking some time to understand why you don't prioritise relationships and exploring the practical things you can do to address that.

It's also worth saying that going through this process and analysing what went wrong won't always end up with you ploughing ahead. Sometimes we learn that it is time to give up and try something completely different. I stopped doing gymnastics at around the age of 14. It was at a time when British gymnastics was not what it is today and there wasn't really the funding that we've seen in recent years. Back then, you either made it to the Olympics by the age of 16 or you didn't, and I knew by the time I was hitting my teens that I wasn't going to make the grade. I went through puberty and couldn't lift my body weight in the same way any more, so I had to find something else in my life. I did some athletics and tennis, as well as trying out a variety of other sports. So, failure doesn't just help to move you closer to your destination, it also tells you when it is time to change your path entirely.

Turning the cycle of reflection and learning from failure into a habit, and recognising the benefits of failure instead of fearing it, won't just benefit you in the long term, it's helpful for those around you, too. Psychologist Kyla Haimovitz, while at Stanford University, found that parents' beliefs about whether failure is good or bad guide how their children think about their own intelligence, so making sure you have a healthy relationship with not getting things right is vital not only for your own well-being but for your children's as well. Let them know when you've messed up and tell them what you've learned from it – on a basic level, that might be telling them why dinner is burned and what you did wrong and what you've learned and will do right next time. Take frying an egg . . . stick with me here. If the pan is too hot and you burn it, the failure provides the knowledge that the pan shouldn't be as hot next time. That's a very simple example, but there's been an action, some reflection and a plan going forward of what to change whenever you next fry an egg.

Micro failures like this can provide a blueprint for how to deal with bigger failures, and you can pass this blueprint on to your kids at a young age. You run out of milk – you pop to the shops, get some more and remember to buy a bigger carton next time you go to the supermarket. These micro failures are an incredibly effective way of teaching kids how to extract the lessons from things that go wrong. But also share with them some of your bigger mistakes – not only can they learn from the things that have gone wrong in your life, but it shows them that it is OK to try and to fail. There's nothing to be ashamed of. In fact, it is an excellent recipe for success.

* * *

Sometimes, however, it can be difficult to identify why something went wrong and no amount of self-assessment will be enough on its own to show you how to fix the problem. This is where feedback comes in. Feedback is one of the best tools we have to improve our performance, and how we respond to it after failure is vital for growth. When I was a teacher, there was constant feedback: appraisals from bosses, feedback from colleagues and pupils, league tables that showed how the kids were doing. When I stepped out of the classroom and started to work with the newspaper and publishing industries, the feedback was pretty much non-existent. Lots of businesses work in that way, but it's not something I was accustomed to.

It was so alien to me that, when one of my editors at the daily newspaper for which I had been writing for around a year invited me for lunch, I was convinced she was going to fire me. I'd not really heard much from her and so presumed the worst. Having not had constant feedback when I was previously used to it made me sure I'd failed in a spectacular way. Without feedback, I'd let my mind wander towards negative thoughts, and I automatically presumed the very worst. I was adamant she was taking me to a restaurant to deliver the bad news so that I wouldn't shout and scream, and I barely slept the entire week leading up to it. Needless to say, when I got there, after some small talk, she told me she was delighted with my work, and we spent a very enjoyable lunch catching up. This episode showed just how important feedback is to me.

Ask yourself who you get feedback from and what that feedback looks like. Look at as many situations as you can – does your spouse or partner ever give you feedback? Do your kids? Do your colleagues or bosses? What does that feedback consist of and what form does it take? How does it make you feel about yourself? Are you open to it, or do you go on the defensive? No one really enjoys having a spotlight shone on their shortcomings, but if you can get over your bruised ego and start to see that feedback genuinely given by someone who knows what they're talking about is just constructive criticism that will help you to do better next time, you will begin to welcome it with open arms.

Feedback is one of the best tools we have to improve our performance.

Actively seeking out, receiving and digesting feedback, even if it's not what you want to hear in that moment, is often easier if it comes from a trusted source. If your loving partner or the boss who you really respect tells you where you went wrong, it can sink in more and is more likely to prompt a change in behaviour. So try to find people in your life who you can look to for honest and helpful feedback. If nothing else, an outside perspective can help you to reach your own conclusions about where you went wrong.

* * *

We've talked about embracing failure because of the opportunity it provides for learning and improvement, but the final thing I want to say about failure is that it can also increase drive and passion.

I worked at some pretty underprivileged schools in my teaching career – schools in difficult areas with high unemployment, social problems and a lack of equality. On paper they were deemed as 'failing schools', and yet at every single one of those schools there were plenty of kids who were using their circumstances as motivation to change them. They didn't like their lives, they didn't like the poverty they and their families lived in, so they used it as a fire in their bellies to try hard in school, get good grades and lift themselves out of poverty.

If you make excuses for what has gone wrong, you won't address it and you'll struggle to use it as a driver, but if you see your failure or the difficulties you are facing as a reason to try harder, you'll find the tools and the inspiration you need to keep moving forward.

Following my cancer diagnosis, I could have stayed in a puddle of my own tears for months, years even (don't get me wrong, you'll find me there sometimes), but my drive to make my life – however long or short it might be – a rich and well-lived one is what spurs me on every single day. I might not be able to do much about my body failing, but I've found other successes I can celebrate. And they are what keep me going.

Whatever difficulties you are facing, even if they are something you feel is immovable right now, move towards success however you can, in any direction – step by step, minute by minute, day by day – and you will soon see that your failures helped you to get where you wanted to go.

'I'm not afraid of storms, for I'm learning how to sail my ship'

Louisa May Alcott

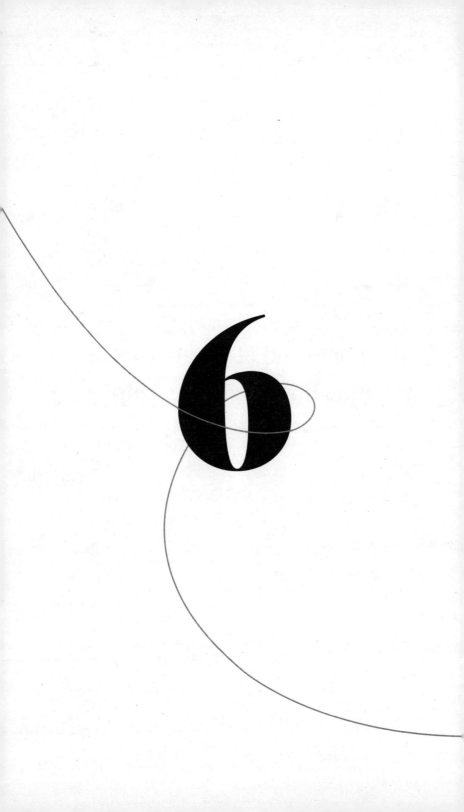

it's time to get
gritty

'Never give up, for that is just the place and time that the tide will turn'

Harriet Beecher Stowe

In my first year of teaching, when I was in my early twenties, I came across this quote often said to be by Eleanor Roosevelt, the longest-serving first lady of the United States: 'The future belongs to those who believe in the beauty of their dreams.' It was my first job and I wanted to impress, so I spent hours in the reprographics room after work printing the quote onto little cards and laminating them so that I could give one to every single child in the school to keep with them. I thought that quote was like a spell. If you dreamed big and believed in those dreams, they'd come true.

Looking back, I don't know whether I'm impressed at my enthusiasm or incredulous I thought it was that simple – that if you wanted something badly enough, it would happen. If that was the case, I would have cured my cancer and I'd be a billionaire. I do think there is an element of truth expressed by the quote – we all need to give space to our dreams, because it's only by letting our imagination conjure up a future life for ourselves that we can understand what we want and begin to see how we might make it happen. But, ultimately, it will only be possible if you show up and approach things with resilience and self-belief and commitment.

You would have thought I'd have known better, really, as I learned about the power of determination and putting in the hard work from a young age. When I was in the national gymnastics programme, I trained as much as 30 hours a week. It was instilled in us that hard work would produce results and that you had to be incredibly disciplined with what you were doing. What I learned from gymnastics has stayed with me for the rest of my life. It makes me laugh now to think about what I was able to achieve. I was pushing my body to the absolute limits as a really young child. Whether that was healthy is a totally different debate. But when it came to instilling in me a belief that I could achieve something if I practised over and over, it was invaluable, and it set me up to be able to do things later in life that I didn't think were possible.

When I was 12, I broke my ankle. I was working on performing sequences of backflips on the beam and my hand slipped on my second flip. As I fell, my feet crashed into the side of the apparatus. Because I was already in rotation, my body carried on and propelled me from the side of the beam, and I broke my ankle when I landed.

Once I'd recovered, I was utterly petrified to get back on the beam, and I basically had to start again from scratch. In order to rebuild, I had to go back to square one. It would have been easy to give up and succumb to my anxiety about hurting myself again, but I loved gymnastics and wanted to be successful at it. I had to find my grit and determination to keep going.

We also had a mantra that sums up grit for me. At the end of a session, you'd never want your last dismount or your last move of whatever it was that you were working on to be a bad one. This meant there were occasions when you would go half an hour or more over your gym session. It was a mental state of saying to yourself, 'No, I can do this.' And it set you up really well for the next time. Even if you'd done a hundred bad moves, if you ended on one good one, you would be more likely to come back in and say, 'Actually, it's OK. I can do it again.' It was about keeping going until you got the result you wanted, and it took a whole lot of grit when all you wanted to do was go home and rest.

Grit, to me, means the outright refusal to yield, to keep picking yourself up again, to always find a way to persevere and keep going, and it is vital to living like there's no tomorrow. And since being diagnosed with incurable cancer, I have had to call on grit time and time again. I've had several allergic reactions to chemotherapy and, as a result, it became psychologically very difficult to do the treatment that was so necessary to my survival. On one occasion, I had a particularly serious anxiety attack when I was undergoing chemo. Medically I was fine, but I was utterly sure I would die. I was convinced that was it – D-Day had arrived and I was about to shuffle off. Fortunately, I managed to persevere and complete the dose.

While most people would avoid something if it induced that level of trauma, I had no option but to go back and get more chemotherapy a few weeks later. I really can't overstate how much I didn't want to. Even though I knew my life would be shorter if I didn't show up, it was still so difficult to drive there, undo my seatbelt and enter the hospital. It was life-saving treatment, but such was my anxiety about suffering another allergic reaction that it took everything I had, every ounce of grit I could muster, to get it done. I'm guessing most cancer patients have felt like this at some point – when the treatment seems worse than the disease, and it takes a huge amount of resolve to keep going.

Grit means the outright refusal to yield, and it is vital to living like there's no tomorrow.

I suppose you could say that my childhood gymnastics and the career I loved so much in teaching helped to make me a determined person who didn't like to give up. But, since my diagnosis, grit has become an even bigger part of who I am, and I'm now able to apply it to other areas of my life – cancer is godawful, and there's no way anyone wants the bloody thing, but it's revealed a level of grit and perseverance I didn't know I had. When the chips were down, I found a way to keep living. Facing up to the things I wanted to do least was the only way I could do that. If you've ever been in a similar situation, you'll know that when you dig deep, those are the times you gain the most, when you're most proud of yourself.

* * *

When I was a teacher, I used to lead all kinds of teacher development and training in different schools. I also liked to recommend books about mindset, leadership and development to people who were interested in learning more, like *Mindset* by Carol Dweck, *Bounce* by Matthew Syed and particularly *Grit* by psychologist Angela Duckworth, who wanted to understand why some people succeed and others fail. Her research led her to study groups with very different goals and markers of success – for example, West Point military academy graduates and children at spelling competitions in America. Here, she found the greatest indicators for success were less about innate talent and more about passion, perseverance and conscientiousness. 'Talent distracts us from something that is at least as important, and that is effort,' she wrote. She and her colleagues labelled this trait 'grit', which they ultimately came to define as 'passion and perseverance for long-term goals'.

No matter how many times you fail or get knocked down, grit means that you'll get back up again. It means that you'll dedicate the time and effort you need to become better and get what you want, and not get way-laid along the way. It's one of the X factors when it comes to success and living your life to the fullest. It means that you don't give up in the face of adversity or at the first obstacle in your way. If you've identified your failures and know what caused them, like we discussed in the previous chapter, grit is what will help you to put them right, allowing you to persevere and keep going when things get tough.

I once met a young Eton graduate who was a first-generation refugee from Somalia. David had arrived in London as a baby with his parents, and he and his four siblings lived in a tower block in an area of London with a high crime rate. David attended the biggest comprehensive in the area. It was a good school, and the grades its pupils achieved were better than you might expect given the difficulties they faced – English was often their second language, and they generally didn't have access to computers or printers at home. David couldn't attend many clubs because he had to be home after school to look after his younger siblings. But he dreamed big. He found out Eton had a sixth-form scholarship for children like him and, with help from his teachers, he applied. He was shortlisted and interviewed and received a conditional offer to do his A levels there as long as he got top marks across the board in his GCSEs.

That summer was one of the warmest on record – the sun shone in London, and David's many friends constantly called by, asking him to come out and play football in the park, but he kept his focus on his studies. He also kept his offer letter by his bed so he could see it every night before he went to sleep and remind himself of what he would be passing up if he didn't dedicate himself to those exams. He told himself he needed to persevere, sacrifice and be conscientious in the short term so he could reach his goals in the long term.

David went to Eton, got straight As in his A levels and, a few years later, was accepted to the University of Oxford.

David has grit, bucketloads of it. He knew at a very young age that unless he put in the hours and made sacrifices, he

No matter how many times you fail or get knocked down, grit means that you'll get back up again.

wouldn't get the opportunities in life that he so desperately wanted. Many of us don't reach our goals like David did because we're not willing to keep going when things get tough. But we'll only get what we want with work and perseverance.

In her book, Angela Duckworth describes the formula that she has come up with to describe this kind of grit:

$$TALENT \times EFFORT = SKILL$$
$$SKILL \times EFFORT = ACHIEVEMENT$$

'Talent is how quickly your skills improve when you invest effort,' she explains. 'Achievement is what happens when you take your acquired skills and use them.' In other words, without effort, your talent is just what you could have been capable of if you'd tried; skill can only get you where you want it to if you put in effort. David was academically gifted, but he tried hard and made sacrifices to get where he wanted to go. He persevered in the face of a long hot summer when he could have been derailed. He dug deep despite being a teenager who wanted to play football with his friends.

I'm sure most of us can think of a similar situation when we had to find grit we didn't know we had. Maybe you resat exams you failed just so you could get into the college or university you wanted to go to despite being a year behind your friends. Maybe you kept going with a new exercise regime even when it got tough and you didn't feel like you were making any progress. Maybe you went for that promotion again after having been told you didn't make the grade the year before.

Something like this happened to me during my teaching career. I was an assistant head but wanted to make the next step up to deputy head. Although the two roles sound kind of similar, they are, in fact, quite different. A deputy head has legal responsibility for a school in the absence of a head teacher, and you need a special qualification – the National Professional Qualification for Headship. I knew I could do the job, but whenever I received feedback, I was told I was rushing it and wasn't ready. Rather than shrinking into myself and taking the feedback negatively, I worked harder and made sure that people's perceptions of me matched my ability to do the job. I had to swallow my pride and overcome the feelings of rejection, make some sacrifices and keep my eyes on the prize. And it helped that I was so passionate about the ultimate goal, as this is another important aspect of grit. The next time I went for the promotion, I got it.

While most of us have probably shown grit like this at some point in our lives, not all of us can call on it whenever we want to. The question is: how do we harness grit and employ it in everyday life to make it part of who we are? How do we make it more likely that when we are distracted, derailed or thrown a curveball, we can dust ourselves down and get back to where we want to be as soon as possible?

It obviously helps if you are pursuing what interests you. If you are going after something that's not right for you or chasing a goal imposed on you by the expectations of others, it's definitely going to be harder to stay the course. Really wanting it and having passion for what you do are key ingredients.

Passion has a specific meaning in Duckworth's theory. When it comes to grit, she says it's not intense emotions that count – passion in this context is more about having overarching goals and pursuing them consistently over a long period of time, as you only pursue things over the long term if you really care about them. Duckworth refers to these as 'top-level goals', or goals that are ends unto themselves rather than the lower-level goals that are a means to an end. As we saw in Chapter 3, living a long happy life with cancer is for me a top-level goal, whereas drinking a healthy smoothie is a lower-level goal that helps me to achieve my main one.

Each of us will have something that motivates and engages us – applying effort in this aspect of our lives is much more likely to reap rewards than trying to win *Bake Off* if you hate cake. If your goal doesn't inspire you, it might be the wrong one for you. The things you are working towards should have a meaning to them, even if that meaning is only relevant to you.

But whatever it is, you need to practise. *Outliers*, the book by the author and journalist Malcolm Gladwell, helped to popularise the '10,000-hour rule' – the gist of which is that 10 years of practising 1,000 hours a year is required to reach excellence in any given pursuit, whether that be elite sportsperson or concert pianist. The idea was taken up in Matthew Syed's bestselling book *Bounce*, but with an important proviso – there's no point doing 10,000 hours of practice badly. Talent does still play a part, and the effort we put in needs to be focused and realistic – most of us are not going to become professional tennis players, even with 10,000 hours of practice. And particularly not if that practice doesn't stretch and challenge us, revealing our weaknesses so we can actively work on them. But the fact remains that it is difficult to get good at something – from riding a skateboard to being an impressive public speaker – without putting in the hours. There's no such thing as overnight success, despite what Hollywood might want us to believe. A young footballer who makes their Premier League debut and scores in their first match might be an unknown name until that night, but they will have spent thousands of hours practising, staying late after training and getting there early, and working on summoning their grit when they hit hurdles along the way.

Those hurdles will be different for everyone, and they can also change over time. When I was growing up, I was never particularly nervous about public speaking. If someone asked me to say a few words at a family event, I'd have no problem standing up in front of everyone and talking. But when I first had to speak to an audience of people in a professional capacity, I was a nervous wreck. I was shaking so much at my first assembly that the head noticed and had to coach me to get over my nerves. With practice, I did, and it got to the point that it was second nature to me. It was a case of accepting some help, digging deep and practising until speaking in a professional context started to feel like quite a normal thing to do. I experienced something similar when I embarked on my media career to raise awareness of my illness. In retrospect, spreading the word about bowel cancer on TV and radio was a natural extension of my passion and talent for education, but when I made my first live appearance, on *BBC Breakfast*, I was so nervous at the thought of millions of people watching me. But I got through it as best I could, and each subsequent live interview or podcast made me a little bit more practised in communicating in this way.

The things you are working towards should have a meaning to them.

Optimistic or positive self-talk has also been shown to be an important part of cultivating perseverance and grit.

The US military teaches its recruits this and professional athletes use it as part of their training. At its core, it's as simple as saying, 'You've got this' when things get tough. Research suggests that people who use optimistic self-talk have reduced stress levels and are more likely to succeed. If this sounds like poppycock, I promise you it's not. Think about the number of times you've told yourself that you can't do something, it's too hard or you're not smart enough, and how often that language has become a self-fulfilling prophecy – that's pessimistic or negative self-talk, which we often direct at ourselves without giving it a second thought. Optimistic self-talk turns this process on its head.

I definitely would have struggled more with a particularly challenging task I signed up to a couple of years ago without harnessing the power of positive self-talk! Back in 2019, I took part in Tri January, a campaign by British Triathlon to get people into the sport. As I've said, exercise has always been a really important part of my approach to cancer – it's good for keeping my anxiety in check, as well as for preparing for and recovering from some major operations. I was therefore really up for helping them to promote their campaign – but with just one problem: I'm petrified of swimming in open water. Even though I received advice and training from Olympic gold medallist Rebecca Adlington, when I entered the freezing cold water to do the swim part of the triathlon, in one of the lakes in Roundhay Park in Leeds, I just froze and thought, 'I can't breathe.'

It was a triathlon for beginners, so the swim was only 400 metres, which I knew I could do because I'd done it many times in a swimming pool. But when you're standing in a murky lake and the water's 12°C, all logic goes out of the window. I wanted to be anywhere else than there, but BBC Sport had cameras at the event and I thought I'd be letting people down if I gave up. I positioned myself next to the safety boat and said to myself, 'Deborah, you can do this.' And I repeated this mantra for the whole 400 metres. 'You can do this. You can do this.'

Afterwards, I promised myself I would never, ever swim in open water again, because I hated it so much. *I absolutely hated it.* I knew I'd hate it before I started, and I still hated it after I'd finished. But I did it. And I did it because of positive self-talk. It gave me the grit and determination not to fail at something. I just had to tell myself I could do it. And it's now the medal I treasure the most, alongside the one I got for running the London Marathon.

Finally, it helps if you can surround yourself with people who have the same goals and a similar passion for them as you do. Teachers know that when a new kid arrives at school, they're very likely to behave like the kids they hang around with, so we encourage all children to choose their friendships wisely. Similarly, when you join a sports group or club, you often end up adopting their training ethic. If you find others like you with similar goals, ideals and processes, you're more likely to stick to your target and even get there a bit faster. Support, encouragement and a healthy dose of competition go a long way to increasing your grit.

* * *

If grit is about persevering in the pursuit of long-term goals, then where does resilience fit into the picture? Grit and resilience are, of course, similar, most obviously in that they both encapsulate an ability to keep going when things get tough, but they are also distinct in a number of important ways.

In psychology, resilience is a trait that allows you to respond to the challenges in your life in a proactive way, employing skills and strategies that help you to cope and recover more effectively. But it's not just about being able to cope in the moment; resilience is also about coming out of the other side of adversity a stronger and more resourceful person, thereby increasing your ability to deal with the next difficult situation you might face. The unpredictability of life is a given; we can expect to be tripped up from time to time. But the question is, how quickly can you get over a stressful time, regain your equilibrium and refocus your energies on where you want to go next? And, once the immediate stresses caused by the situation have passed, can you continue to grow and use those negative experiences as fuel, or at least a learning opportunity, for the future? Resilience can develop over time, particularly if you've faced challenges and overcome them.

There are a number of theories about what makes someone resilient, and where their resilience comes from. The qualities said to be present in a resilient person fall under two broad headings: a strong sense of self and good interpersonal skills.

Expectation of success in life is a little like positive self-talk. By remaining positive, it allows you to focus on the outcome you want and makes it less likely you'll feel derailed or distracted by the possibility of things not going your way. At the same time, believing in yourself and those talents you worked hard to turn into skills promotes a sense of agency and control over the things that happen to you. In other words, rather than making excuses or claiming that large external forces, such as fate, are to blame, a self-confident individual believes they are capable of tackling any problems that arise. If you have good insight into what motivates you, how you feel about things and how this affects you, as well as feeling comfortable admitting both your strengths and your weaknesses, you will invariably find that you are better placed to withstand life's challenges. This self-knowledge and sense of personal identity also brings with it a greater sense of meaning and purpose in your life, which makes you much less likely to give up when faced with adversity – after all, it's easier to keep going if you feel that what you are doing is worthwhile.

Resilient people are determined, persistent, maintain a sense of balance and sustain effort. They plan for the future, but they are also flexible and can adapt when faced with challenges, as well as accepting setbacks along the way. It is much harder to be resilient if you allow yourself to become overwhelmed by negative thoughts or resort to destructive actions whenever something doesn't go the way you hoped. If you are more open to positive emotions and able to exhibit some self-control, such as an ability to resist strong impulses and delay gratification, you are more likely to be resilient in the face of difficulties. Similarly, in times of stress, you are more likely to be resilient if you have tried-and-tested coping strategies that you can call on. Some examples of these might include turning to others for help, boosting your own state of mind by helping others, coming up with potential solutions to problems ahead of time and reframing adversity – for example, by seeing the irony or funny side of a difficult situation. If you can express your feelings clearly and honestly, this allows you to examine your thoughts, emotions, motivations and actions and develop your resilience.

It's also really important to take care of your body by eating well, getting enough sleep and exercising. If you don't feel physically well, it's hard to find the mental fortitude to be resilient in the face of challenges. And don't mask stress with negative coping mechanisms, such as alcohol and drugs, over- or undereating, gambling or excessive sleeping. I'm not suggesting you have to live a holier-than-thou existence, and it's good to let your hair down from time to time – after all, I've been known to like a glass of wine now and again! – but you can't come to depend on potentially destructive outlets.

Resilience allows you to respond to the challenges in your life in a proactive way.

Although honesty and taking responsibility for all of your actions is vital, resilience is not all on you. Relying on the support of others is also really important – something I've come to appreciate more and more as my health has deteriorated. This is why having access to social support aids a person's ability to be resilient, while becoming isolated can damage it. I'm sure you'll have seen reports in the news about the 'loneliness epidemic' and our increasing understanding that lack of social connection – for example, among the elderly or during the Covid-19 pandemic – has a profoundly negative effect on people's physical and mental well-being. So, addressing loneliness is not just about improving people's quality of life – it is an important issue that needs to be at the centre of public-health policy.

Finding people who are going through the same thing as you can be really powerful. I wouldn't wish bowel cancer on anyone, but forming a support network or community of people who can understand what you're talking about without you having to spell out every detail is liberating. I often get calls from friends, or friends of friends, asking me to talk to someone they know who has been diagnosed with bowel cancer. I'm obviously not a doctor, and I can't give them medical advice, but I do know how scary it is. When you are first diagnosed, you think you're the only person out there who has ever gone through this until you discover that there are sadly thousands of other people who are going through it too. I think, until that point, you feel totally isolated and you don't know what to do. When you realise you're not alone, it gives your resilience a real boost.

It might not come easily to you, but the more sociable, open, gracious and affable you can be, the more friendships and connections you will make, and the greater your support network will be. But the size of your network is less important than the strength of the bonds you have with people, so even if you are more of an introvert at heart, it's always worth trying to make meaningful personal connections in your life.

Being open to expressing your emotions makes it easier to connect with people on a genuine level, which in turn allows for more meaningful relationships to form. In this way, being able to call on people you trust helps you to be more resilient. And empathy for other people leads to stronger relationships too. Being unselfish, altruistic and generally caring about the welfare of others means those people are generally more likely to want to be in relationships with you and help you out when you need it.

So, resilience is very much about you as an individual, but it's also about your relationships with the people around you. Understanding this is an important first step towards being able to deal with anything that life throws at you.

* * *

There are practical things you can do to be a more resilient person. Some people more naturally possess some of the attributes that help underpin resilience, and therefore find that it comes more easily to them. But that doesn't mean everyone else should just give up. Having had to scrape myself off the floor more times than I can tell you in the last few years, I really believe it's something that can be developed and learned. And the American Psychological Association (APA) agrees with me: 'resilience involves behaviors, thoughts, and actions that anyone can learn and develop'.

Cognitive behavioural therapy (often just known as CBT) is a type of therapy that helps you to turn around negative thought processes that might be undermining your resilience and to develop the skills to cope with problems when they occur. But even without undertaking formal therapy, there are a range of things you can do to help improve on the natural store of resilience you already possess. The APA has produced a helpful ten-point list of things you can try:

1. Make connections.
2. Avoid seeing crises as insurmountable problems.
3. Accept that change is a part of living.
4. Move towards your goal.
5. Take decisive actions.
6. Look for opportunities for self-discovery.
7. Nurture a positive view of yourself.
8. Keep things in perspective.
9. Maintain a hopeful outlook.
10. Take care of yourself.

I promise you that resilience isn't some kind of superpower. People say to me, 'I don't know how you stay so positive.' And I don't all the time. But I wholeheartedly believe that most of us would be surprised by just how resilient we can be when the chips are really down. Regardless, I've learned that resilience and grit are traits we can actively cultivate to help us achieve the things we want. We don't have to wait for some disaster to befall us to find out what we are really made of.

'No grit, no pearl'

Anonymous

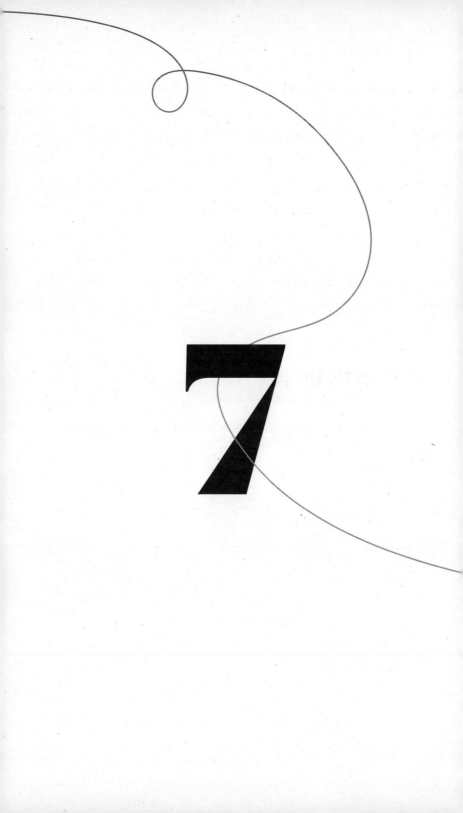

the courage
to face your fears

'You gain strength, courage and confidence by every experience in which you really stop to look fear in the face. You are able to say to yourself, "I have lived through this horror. I can take the next thing that comes along"'

Eleanor Roosevelt

W hat's your most embarrassing moment? One of mine was in Karen Millen in Covent Garden when I was 24. Though whenever I think about it now, it's not with shame or mortification. I can recall exactly the feeling of being abjectly terrified – experiencing a level of fear that overrode any sense of, 'Oh dear, this is a bit embarrassing.' I genuinely thought I was about to drop dead.

I was in the changing rooms, in a hot, stuffy underground cubicle, in the middle of trying on a dress I thought I wanted for work, when suddenly a wave of utter, immense, breathtaking fear overcame me. As anyone who has had a panic attack will attest, they tend to come out of nowhere. So I was completely blindsided. My lungs felt like they'd ceased to function, and I had the urge to run, to try to put some distance between me and the way I was feeling. I wanted to run out of my body, if at all possible, but at the very least I knew that I physically just had to move ... The problem was I hadn't yet put my clothes back on. So, dressed only in my underwear, I simply grabbed what I had been wearing and ran out of the shop and slap bang into Covent Garden during a busy weekday lunchtime. It was only that crisp, first inhalation of fresh air that made me realise I was standing in the middle of central London in my undercrackers.

Nearby shoppers had stopped to see if I was the next street theatre act. My mind was still flooded with panic, but I managed to find the sense to put my clothes back on. And I ran. I ran across Waterloo Bridge as fast as I could back to the station, eventually onto a train and then home to Woking. I distinctly recall sitting on the train with my Nokia phone texting my mum: 'Don't like central London. Pick up at station in 20 mins?' I then played *Snake* (there's an early noughties reference for you!) the rest of the way to numb my inner 'I'm going to die from not being able to breathe' thoughts.

I've lived with anxiety most of my life. I've been through periods of incredibly frequent, crippling panic attacks that saw me unable to drive a car and rendered me

too scared to walk down a busy street or even to go outside. I ended up in A&E on numerous occasions in my
twenties – such was the severity of what I was feeling, I
could only think that I was having a heart attack. I often
woke up in the middle of the night already in the grip of
an episode, an overwhelming surge of adrenalin coursing
through me, my body numb, feeling completely unable to
move. I believed all the physiological symptoms I was
feeling were messages that my body was dying. The great
irony, of course, being that when I was younger and not
facing death, my fear of it was so uncontrolled that quite
often it stopped me from living. I stayed at home when I
should have been out enjoying myself; I missed holidays
because of my fear of flying.

I would have loved to have been able to take a pill or
push a button and have my crippling anxiety disappear,
but if you have been through anything remotely like
this, or have been there trying to support someone who
has, you'll know it's far from simple. I tried prescription
drugs, but they just made me feel so numb that I couldn't
really feel anything. I've had lots of one-on-one therapy
and CBT with varying results, including some limited
success. But nothing really worked in the long term. So,
as with so many hard, sad or unpleasant things in life, I
had no choice but to try to learn from what I was
going through and find a way forward. I saw a pattern
emerge. My anxiety would build over seemingly nothing,

manifesting in physical ways: panic attacks, shortness of breath. I'd then have to see the GP to get the symptoms checked out for some reassurance. I'd then be OK for a while before the whole thing would start over again.

Do you know what finally 'cured' me? The worst happened and my fear was realised – I was told I had incurable cancer and that I would die. I had no choice any more; I had to look my biggest fear straight in the eye.

I'm not, of course, suggesting for one second that if you have panic attacks there is nothing to be done unless you receive an incurable cancer diagnosis, which will sort you right out. There are many other ways that might help – from CBT and other talking therapies to mindfulness and relaxation techniques – and I would urge you to keep trying to find a solution, because no one should have to live with that level of daily anxiety. But honestly, for me, that diagnosis did something that nothing else had.

Considering I'd spent so much of my life in a heightened state of panic, to the point where I'd once run around one of London's main tourist districts in my pants, on paper I could have – and

I had to look my biggest fear straight in the eye.

perhaps should have – had an absolute breakdown; the panic attack to end all panic attacks. But what actually happened was the oddest, most unexpected thing: my anxiety levels dropped. Of course, there were and still are utter lows and sometimes I feel panic at scans, blood tests or treatments, but these are real events that come with the risk of pain, discomfort and bad news.

When I was forced to confront what I'd spent 20 years worrying about, something shifted in me. I had no choice but to overcome my fear and anxiety about death. I had no choice because I didn't want to die that day, the next day, the next week or the next year. I could either curl up into a ball and await death, or I could keep living in whatever way I chose until the inevitable happened. I had to face my worst-case scenario, but in *having* to, I realised I *could*. My self-doubt disappeared bit by bit. I didn't realise my strength until I had no choice; my fight to live was stronger than my fear of death.

* * *

People often tell me, very kindly, that they think I'm brave. But I don't think of myself like that. When you find yourself in a horrible situation like mine, you don't have a lot of choice but to just get on with it. I think I'm only doing what any of us would do. It comes down in large part to motivation. You never think, 'I'm going to keep going because I'm brave.' You keep going because you've got something to keep going for.

One Friday, I was in hospital and my interventional radiologist had to put in an emergency drain to help clear my bile duct. It was the classic situation just before the weekend in a hospital – everything is rushed, so there was no time for me to be sedated or to receive any of the nice drugs that make it all OK. He just had to go ahead and put the drain in, and afterwards he said, 'Deborah, you're more hardcore than any of us give you credit for. You didn't even flinch.'

I said, 'Well, we just had to get the job done.'

'I know, but I have had grown men cry on me!'

To me, courage is when you don't want to do something but you do it anyway. It's true that there are times when I have made a conscious and active decision to face something that I've found scary. I haven't simply sat back and let the chips fall where they may. I've been positive and made a choice, like when I kept going back for more chemo, even though I had suffered from the allergic reaction and was scared it would happen again. But, at the same time, you often don't really have a choice. When people tell me I'm brave, my response is usually, 'What else can I do?' If I'm in a medical emergency, I am out of options. If I don't let the doctors do what they need to, I will die. When you don't have a choice, you just close your eyes and grit your teeth and get on with it.

As anyone who has faced a life-changing diagnosis or who has been called on to confront their fears will know, you can be scared and brave at the same time. I am still absolutely petrified a lot of the time. Of course I am. But

I am also able to endure even the scariest things that happen to me.

In early 2022 I almost died following a medical emergency related to my cancer. My treatment had been stopped for four months at the end of 2021 because of a bout of colitis. Despite this, I'd enjoyed a lovely Christmas with my family and was ready to start chemo again in the new year. In the run-up to my appointment at the Marsden on 6 January, I hadn't been feeling great, but I had no idea

Courage is when you don't want to do something but you do it anyway.

how seriously ill I was. A blood test showed that my liver function was dangerously out of kilter, and further investigation revealed that the tumour around my bile duct had grown during the gap in treatment and was now blocking it. Thankfully, it was operable, and I was booked in for the next day.

That evening, at around six o'clock, I started to feel very unwell. I ran to the bathroom and began to vomit large volumes of fresh blood and clots. It was terrifying. I was extremely dizzy and on the verge of passing out, but I managed to call an ambulance. I could barely get the words out to the emergency call handler at the other end of the phone. I was able to give my name and address, but I couldn't say much more about my condition or situation. I was simply pleading for help.

My husband Seb arrived home to find me in this state, and it's just as well he did. The controller on the phone proceeded to tell him that it would be at least 30 minutes until an ambulance would reach us, so he picked me up, bundled me in the car and sped me to Chelsea and Westminster Hospital. On the way, I was just about holding on to consciousness. I couldn't stop thinking that if the A&E staff didn't know my complex medical history, they might presume I was beyond saving, so I somehow managed to phone my interventional radiologist, Nicos Fotiadis, who had operated on me multiple times by that point, to tell him where I was headed. Thankfully, he was on call and told me he would see me there.

On arrival, I was bustled into resuscitation, where the amazing staff on the crash team managed to stabilise me after hours of it being touch and go. The liver failure had caused my portal vein – the main blood vessel that drains blood from the spleen and gastrointestinal tract to the liver – to rupture, and swollen veins in my oesophagus, known as varices, were bleeding. Both needed to be dealt with if I was to stand any chance of survival. The portal vein was operated on that night by Nicos – I was awake throughout the procedure as I was too weak to take a general anaesthetic. Then, the following morning, the ruptured varices were repaired. Over the following days, I had an allergic reaction to some of my drugs, but they soon managed to find ones that my weakened body could tolerate, and the blocked bile duct, the initial cause of my problems, was also fixed. I spent ten days in hospital not knowing if I would ever leave.

Following the trauma of this event, I was utterly lost again and didn't know what to do with myself. I didn't trust my body, which is very common when you've been through health trauma or have a serious, life-threatening illness. You feel scared to do anything in case it exacerbates your symptoms. You worry that something you have done might have caused a particular incident. You ask yourself questions like, 'If I eat this, is it going to make my cancer worse?'; 'If I exercise, am I going to make myself really tired?' You can second-guess every movement and action, with the result that you are then too scared to step outside your front door. You become trapped in a cycle of vicious thoughts and fear. For me, the only way to break that cycle is to recognise it and move on – that's my strategy. Following my traumatic experience, I forced myself to go out for a walk – that was the first baby step.

That whole experience was terrifying, and it took time for me to come to terms with how close to death I was, but I was able to get to a better place more quickly than I would have been able to when I was first diagnosed. I don't know how to explain it other than I woke up one morning and simply felt a little bit brighter. It was a new day, and I thought, 'I've got too much going on in my life to die now. God, it will be such a faff. There's so much sorting out to do – so much to organise. And I've got things coming up. I've got to write this book, and I've got work stuff. I want to spend quality time with my family. I don't want them to remember me like this. I'd like to get to the south of France again. I do have things to look forward to. Yeah, it would be really annoying if I died.' It's funny how that kind of black humour changed my perspective and made me think, 'Come on, Deborah – let's give it a shot.' It didn't mean my health was suddenly going to improve, but I see now that's a kind of courage, because sometimes the hardest challenge is learning to live again, especially when everything was telling me that what I was facing was almost insurmountable. But if you've got a 1 per cent chance of living, that's something to hold on to. A 1 per cent chance is better than nothing.

However, the challenges kept coming. My cancer had advanced to the point that it essentially meant my liver had stopped working, and the next four months or so were mainly spent in hospital. I hit rock bottom so many times, and I don't know how often I said to myself, 'I don't know how to do this. I don't know how anyone can do this. My body is smashed.' And then the point came in May 2022 when it was clear that there was nothing more the doctors could do for me. My body was too weak to cope with the interventions needed to turn my liver function around, so my family and I came to the heart-rending decision that it was time for me to go home to my mum and dad's and receive hospice care. Despite always knowing that this day would come, it was still completely devastating to realise that my time was coming to an end. But, even then, I hung on to the fact that I was doing things on my own terms – even at the end of my life.

Sometimes the hardest challenge is learning to live again.

* * *

There is no magic recipe for bravery, no secret weapon for facing up to something you never could have imagined. Being courageous is really hard. People aren't just born brave, and I find it difficult to believe there is anyone who is actually fearless. Even the strongest of us feels fear, though how that manifests itself might be very different for everyone: when I am feeling particularly afraid, my fear manifests itself outwardly with tears, whereas for someone else, fear might be a completely internal process.

I've tried to put a brave face on my situation at times. It's not easy, as I'm rubbish at it, and sometimes I'm not really able to at all. But while I would never tell anyone that they must put on a brave face, I do think there are times when it makes sense – for the sake of your kids, for example. It can also help to prevent your negative thoughts from overwhelming you, stopping the lighter moments of hope and gratitude getting in. And I do think there is something to be said for striving to be carefree and a bit fearless about life, because no one should live their life in fear or worry that they aren't brave enough to face their challenges head-on.

Of course it is hard to be brave when your life hangs in the balance. When you feel like a ticking time bomb and it's catching up with you every single day, it is utterly terrifying. I can feel my body breaking down and, particularly recently, it's becoming hard to live every single day. I don't want people to see me. I don't want people to see my demise, because I find it really heartbreaking myself, let alone what it must be like for them.

But I've found a way to keep going, just like I did when I suffered so badly from anxiety. Then, when the worst happened and I was moved to hospice care, although I was terrified, I found a way to carry on. I thought, 'OK, I'll just get through today.' I'm not sure I've really considered that I was being brave. It's just that the alternative was no picnic either, and if I thought too much about the big picture, I'd have been completely overwhelmed. To me, bravery in that kind of situation is really just continuing to take small steps in the direction that you want to go, even when you're scared. You don't feel like you're doing anything special. You're just doing what you think you need to at that time. It's only when you look back that you appreciate that each of those small steps took courage.

And recognising these small things as being brave has been shown to be a good way of increasing our store of courage for the future. Most psychologists break courage down into three categories: physical, moral and vital. The first of these is probably the most obvious – it is when someone acts in the face of danger, often to help someone else and at risk to themselves. Think of the passer-by who jumps into the river to save a drowning child. Moral courage, on the other hand, is when you do something that you know to be right, even though it might be to your detriment. A good example of this would be a child who stands up to bullies on behalf of a classmate, despite the fact that they themselves could then become the target. The third type of courage is not one you might have thought of before, but it relates to people's ability to cope with long-term illness. This is something that I suppose you could say I have exhibited in the face of cancer, but what is much more interesting to me is that this vital courage is also exhibited by the healthcare professionals who look after people who are unwell, as well as by the friends and family members who support their loved ones through illness.

I'm guessing that most of us if asked to define bravery would think of physical courage first. These are the stories of brave people doing heroic things that we see on the news or read about in novels. Or perhaps your mind turns to a towering figure from history such as Martin Luther King, Jr or Nelson Mandela, both of whom exhibited incredible moral courage to stand up to racial injustice despite the hardships and dangers they faced. These extraordinary acts are by definition rare, and as such we could be forgiven for thinking that courage is in short supply or something that only a few of us possess. However, when you start to think of courage as a state of mind rather than an act, you can see that there are small acts of courage all around us: it is brave to change careers in midlife, to tell someone you love them when you don't know if they will say it back, to create something and put it out into the world knowing that other people might judge it. A shy child going to school for the first time is courageous, as is

Bravery is continuing to take small steps in the direction that you want to go, even when you're scared.

the person who learns to swim even though they are afraid of water. If we recognise these everyday examples of bravery and spend more time bringing them to people's attention, we soon see that there are lots of instances when we, too, have been courageous. That is when we start to realise that we are brave, and that courage is something that we all have inside of

us. And it is this realisation that helps to increase our sense
of courage and ability to be brave when things get tough
or we are made to confront our fears. The truth is, we are
all braver than we realise.

* * *

We all have our fears, and it's important to recognise and
accept that. I think one of the bravest things is learning
how to live in the face of all of life's uncertainties and all
of the things that can go wrong or that can hurt us, physically and mentally. And, of course, fear can be a good
thing. It's there to tell us that we want to live our lives;
that we want to be good at whatever it is we care about.
If you're not a little bit scared sometimes, maybe you
don't really appreciate what's at stake. The key in those
situations is how you control your nerves. Some of the
best public speakers in the world still get anxious. The
most successful sportspeople get nervous before they
compete. And there's nothing wrong with that. In fact,
some people use their nerves as part of their preparation –
if they didn't get a bit scared, it might point to them being
unprepared or not caring enough.

You have to accept and face your fears. There's no
point hiding from what you're scared of, because you
have to acknowledge it if you want to overcome it. Trying
to pretend that you're not scared might be a strategy you

employ occasionally, but it can actually be counter-productive and eventually come back to bite you if it means never facing up to your fears and properly conquering them. So, acknowledge your fears and then move on from them in small steps. That's true courage – to say, 'I'm really scared about what might happen, but I'm going to do it anyway.'

'Each of us must confront our own fears, must come face to face with them. How we handle our fears will determine where we go with the rest of our lives. To experience adventure or to be limited by the fear of it'

Judy Blume

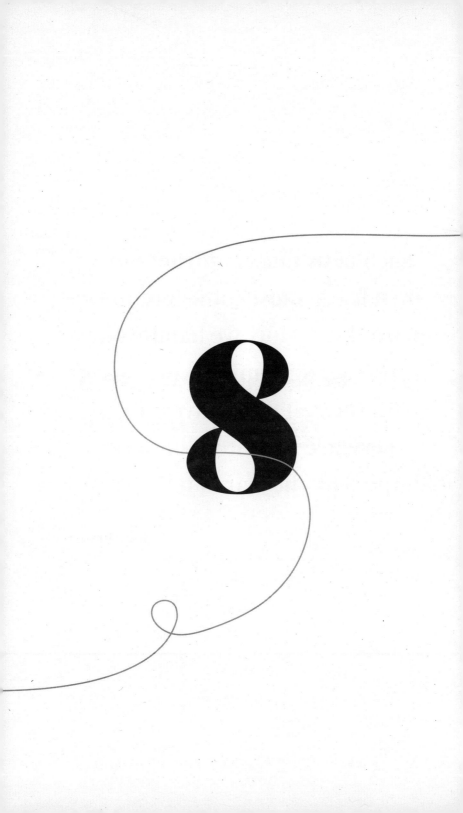

the healing power of
laughter

'I never would have made it if I could not have laughed. It lifted me momentarily out of this horrible situation, just enough to make it liveable'

Viktor Frankl

I've come to learn that having fun and enjoying life is still possible even in the most difficult of situations. In fact, humour plays a massive role in helping me to cope with my cancer. You might not believe me, but I've probably laughed more in the last five years than the previous thirty-five. I think that's reflective of the fact that I have made so much effort to keep life going. Humour is restorative for me, but also for the people around me.

Even in the face of something as shattering as a cancer diagnosis, the world doesn't and can't come to a complete standstill. Your loved ones rally around you, and you're conscious all the time that it changes everything for those people, but life has to go on as well. In this situation, humour offers a bit of protection for those around you.

You can't force laughter on them, but joking gives them permission to smile. Could you imagine if my family had walked around for five years saying, 'Deborah's going to die, Deborah's going to die'? That's not sustainable, and it's just not us – we are a family that loves to smile and joke.

As my health deteriorated from January 2022 onwards, I found myself spending more and more time in hospital. I was having a particularly rough weekend at one point, and the only thing I was able to focus on was whether or not I could fart. Sorry if this is too graphic, but my bowels basically decided not to work – I had colitis and all these other issues.

Humour is restorative for me, but also for the people around me.

So I ended up sharing a post with 400,000 people on Instagram about whether or not I could poo and fart. And then when I finally did fart, I put out a post saying, 'Hallelujah.' I didn't want to focus on how rough I was feeling, so I hid behind humour instead. You have to find the funny side, because sometimes things are so appalling that if you don't laugh, you'll cry – and you do cry anyway, but at least the laughing gets you through those difficult moments.

I had a similar situation earlier this year. It was a silly little thing in the grand scheme of things, but it was definitely a laugh-or-you'll-cry moment. When I was in hospital, because I didn't know if I was going to wake up in a lot of pain, I had to get everything that I might need near me before I went to bed. It was about three o'clock in the morning and I'd just managed to get to sleep after taking a painkiller. About ten minutes later, I kicked an entire jug of water over my sheets. I just lay there for a moment in a massive puddle not doing anything apart from rolling my eyes before I pressed the button for someone to come and help me, thinking, 'Oh my God, this is so Deborah. Just when you eventually get to sleep, you have absolutely cocked up again!' I was in pain, it was the middle of the night and I was having to call on someone to change my bed because I'd left a water jug in the wrong place and decided to roll in the wrong direction. I just had to laugh.

I gravitate more to people who are funny, particularly if they share my sense of humour, which is very silly and very British. I laugh at really juvenile sausage jokes and fart jokes. If it's too clever, I don't get it, to be really honest. Or if it's too highbrow – that's not my kind of thing at all. The other day, I was watching this TV programme at one o'clock in the morning because I was in pain and couldn't sleep. It was one of those terrible middle-of-the-night blooper programmes about the royals being captured on camera getting things wrong, and one of them was wetting themselves listening to a musician who was playing like cats. Not like *Cats* the musical. He was basically making cat sounds to make a tune for some unknown reason, and I was pissing myself. It's really basic stuff like that which I find funny, and in that moment it helped me to forget the pain I was in.

Life can be quite absurd sometimes. You can't predict anything. That's what makes it so interesting but also what makes it so challenging to navigate. Things don't always go to plan or work out how you expect them to, so you have to laugh along the way. Things can get really serious when you're in a situation like mine and everything is a matter of life or death. It's easy to lose sight of humour and the lighter side of life, so sometimes you have to make sure to lighten the mood. If you're shitting yourself every two seconds and have to wear a nappy like a baby, without a bit of humour things could get really depressing really quickly.

I really believe that it's OK to laugh, even in moments of darkness or sorrow. Some of my funniest memories are from the saddest moments of my life. Like when I got absolutely bollocked by my parents for being late to my grandmother's funeral. I'd gone out the night before and drunk too much, and I ended up following the casket down the aisle of the church because I was so late and really hungover. But that's now all I really remember about that funeral, which I think is a positive thing. And it definitely lightened the mood in the moment. The rest of the family were asking where I was and then they saw the coffin come in, with me trailing after it saying, 'Sorry. Sorry. So sorry.' Yes, it was totally disrespectful, but it was also very funny, and I know my grandmother would have laughed her head off. Some people might shy away from humour in a setting like that, but laughter is such a big part of life and needs to be celebrated.

I don't take myself too seriously. People put so much pressure on themselves to be perfect, but we cock up all the time, and you've got to be able to take the piss out of yourself. We're all human at the end of the day, and that includes all of our flaws. It's hard work going through life sometimes, so give yourself a break and have a bit of a laugh – even in the face of death.

You might not expect someone to be telling jokes on their deathbed, but when Rachael Bland was close to the end, she turned to very dark humour as a way of coping with it. I have a GIF that she sent me the day before she died. It's basically two Grim Reapers with the caption, 'See you on the other side!' And she always used to say to me, 'If we died at

It's OK to laugh, even in moments of darkness or sorrow.

the same time, do you think we would get two for one on our funeral flowers?', which would crack me up every time.

When I suffered an oesophageal bleed early in 2022, and it was touch and go whether I'd pull through, some of my deathbed confessions were absolutely hilarious. I basically said to my husband, 'Seb, I know you always think I kissed that guy. I never, ever kissed him.' Of all the things that I could have said in what I thought might be my last moments, whether or not I'd kissed some random bloke at a party when we were much younger was what came to mind. I was also relaying messages to my balding brother that he was starting to look like Prince William and needed to hurry up and propose to his girlfriend (thank God he eventually got the message). It was stuff that was totally irrelevant. It makes me laugh to think that we can be so frivolous at what is supposed to be such a profound moment. And this is one of the benefits of humour when it comes to dealing with adversity – it helps to keep things in perspective and lightens the mood.

Humour has also proven to be an important educational tool. I mean, how do you talk about poo without it? I am a patron of Bowel Cancer UK, and I often found myself explaining to them that if they tried to communicate the symptoms of bowel cancer with some boring bullet points, nobody was going to read them. You need to engage people and then you can tell them the facts. And this is where not taking myself too seriously comes in. One of my earliest Instagram videos was of me dressed up in a six-year-old child's poo-emoji costume running around the woods saying, 'I'm too sexy.' I didn't mean to order a child-sized costume, but when it arrived, I thought, 'What the hell?' You're never going to look stylish dressed up as a poo, and it was only ever supposed to be a way of getting people's attention anyway. This has always been my strategy when it comes to raising awareness of my illness: once I've got you to take notice and have a bit of a laugh, then we can talk about bowel cancer. And this way, hopefully the message will stick.

* * *

Humour has helped me on a daily basis, particularly since my diagnosis. But you don't just need to take my word for it – it has been scientifically proven to be beneficial to your mental and physical health. When I said pissing myself with laughter at royal bloopers helped me to forget about my pain for a bit, it wasn't just wishful thinking on my part. Studies have shown that laughter leads to the release of endorphins, which help the body to deal with pain. In fact, laughter has been shown to be a potentially important part of cancer treatment. One study revealed that patients who were given laughter therapy, doing yoga in which you force yourself to laugh and watching comedy performances, had a greater tolerance for pain. It also helped to reduce their anxiety by decreasing their stress hormones. I'm not sure I fancy laughter yoga all that much personally, but I'm always up for watching a bit of comedy, and it's good to know that there is a biological reason why a few jokes really can help me to feel better.

There are, broadly speaking, two types of humour – on the one hand, there is humour that is more inward looking and helps you to feel better about yourself, and on the other hand there is humour that enhances your relationships with others. Self-enhancing humour is a defence mechanism that helps us to cope with stress and can give us courage when we are faced with adversity, allowing us to feel like we are in control of a difficult situation again so that we can persevere and carry on. If it goes too far, though, it can become self-defeating, with excessively self-disparaging humour sometimes leading to negative feelings, even depression and anxiety. In other words, it's good to take the piss out of yourself sometimes, but only to the point that it feels good and is done with genuine humour, not when you're actually berating yourself and it doesn't feel great any more.

Humour has been scientifically proven to be beneficial to your mental and physical health.

Humour that promotes healthy relationships is referred to by psychologists as being 'affiliative', which simply means that it helps you to make strong personal bonds. It improves other people's sense of well-being, helps to reduce conflict, strengthens ties between people, increases your attractiveness, raises the morale, cohesiveness and identity of group members, and creates an atmosphere of fun and enjoyment. On the negative side, if humour becomes aggressive, it can really harm the person who is the brunt of the joke – something I saw up close in school when kids were bullied by someone who tried to excuse their behaviour by saying that they were 'just having a laugh' – but it's not good for you either, as it can make you angry and hostile. If your idea of a joke is making someone else feel bad about themselves, you'll soon find that people are less likely to want to be your friend. So keep it positive and laugh as often as you can, because it's not just an expression – laughter really is the best medicine at times.

* * *

Humour isn't the only supposedly 'trivial' thing that has really helped me. Since becoming ill, I've been much more likely to look at some flowers and notice how bright and beautiful they are, whereas in the past I'd probably have walked by and not even have clocked them – and a new-found deep appreciation for nature is something that a lot of people who have had life-altering experiences report. The ironic thing, though, is that I've always had another appreciation for beauty, one that you could say is much more frivolous! For me, beauty products and pretty clothes are a massive part of what brings me joy in life.

You might think that if you were coming towards the end of your life, the last thing on your mind would be materialistic items like dresses and make-up. But, oh my God, I'm the total opposite – I can't stop buying stuff!

Looking at pretty dresses, even though I know I might not ever wear them, and sitting at my dressing table with a hundred different lipsticks and beautiful bottles of perfume on it gives me so much joy. I understand if you can't really relate to this at all, as not everyone is into clothes and make-up, and I also appreciate how lucky I am to be able to treat myself like this, but it's my way of looking after myself. And when you feel like your body is falling apart, that is so vital.

Trying to make myself look – and therefore feel – better has been a really important tool for me throughout my illness. I hate seeing myself in the mirror when I'm looking really ill, because I don't want to look like a cancer patient – I want to look like my old self, the one who always dressed to impress. That's why putting on lovely clothes and a bit of lipstick gives me such a boost. So does pampering myself. When I was moved to hospice-from-home care, my brother Ben and sister Sarah would come over to 'babysit' me, and I'd book manicures for everyone and order us all matching pyjamas for no reason other than – why not? Having fun and being a bit silly made us feel like kids again; it was better than any medicine.

One of my best moments in hospital revolved around something that would probably seem absolutely ridiculous to lots of people. In *Sex and the City*, Carrie often wears beautiful Manolo Blahnik shoes, including the classic blue velvet pair with crystals on them. In 2022, Blahnik did an unlikely collaboration with Birkenstock, releasing a pair of flat sandals in blue velvet and crystals. To be clear, for me (and I'm sure many of you would disagree), Birkenstocks are up there with the ugliest shoes you can imagine, but they're also very comfy. I just happened to be awake at four o'clock in the morning when they were being released online, so I said to myself, 'I'm buying a pair.' They were absolutely ludicrous but sold out within half an hour. And they've honestly given me so much joy. Yes, it was a really frivolous purchase, but it was also fun and put a smile on my face.

Sitting at my dressing table with a hundred different lipsticks and beautiful bottles of perfume on it gives me so much joy.

So, my appreciation of beauty might be a bit different from yours, but it's what makes me happy. You might take great pleasure in planting beautiful flowers in your garden, but I always kill my plants. Whatever it is that brings you joy, you never need to apologise for it. Finding a bit of joy, happiness and laughter is what makes life worth living, even when things are at their toughest.

'Think of all the beauty still left around you and be happy'

Anne Frank

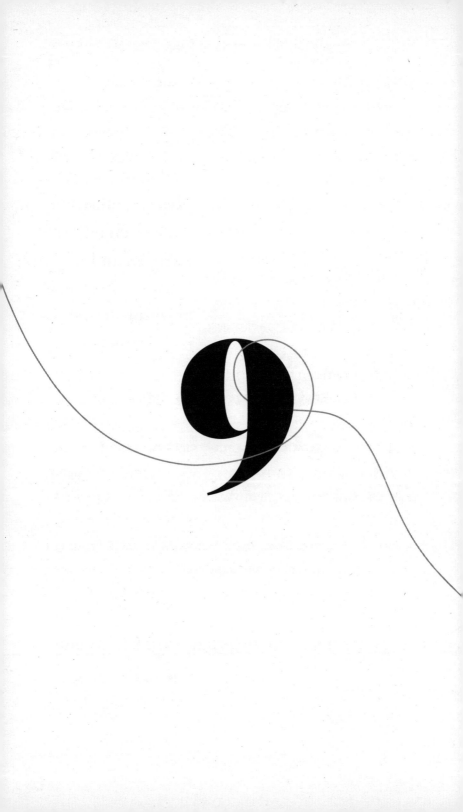

there's always something to be grateful for

'Gratitude is not only the greatest of the virtues but the parent of all others'

Cicero

If you're naturally pessimistic, that's fine, as long as you recognise the fact and try to see the positives a bit more often. Optimistic? Well, that's a blessing. It's true that if you dance in the rain rather than waiting for the storm to pass you will definitely get soaked and perhaps catch cold. Although, on the other hand, I do like dancing, and sometimes getting a bit wet is not the end of the world . . .

My friend Simon taught me this. I met him at university. Simon was born with cystic fibrosis, and he knew he was on borrowed time unless he got a lung transplant. As we all planned what life after university might look like, full of the carelessness of youth, he already knew the value of taking one day at a time – and also how to rock an oxygen tank on the dance floor. When I was diagnosed with cancer, he was the first friend I turned to. He knew exactly what I meant when I said, 'I'm scared.' When everyone else was telling me not to be silly and trying to reassure me that of course I'd have a future, he understood.

His hope arrived in the form of a lung transplant ten years after we left university. He saw life through new glasses. It allowed him to dream of what a future might look like. And then, within a year, his body began to reject the new lungs. In a cruel twist of fate, not only did he know what lay ahead for him, he knew that the flicker of hope he'd been offered had faded to nothing. In fact, it was utterly blown out of the water.

A week before Simon died, I visited him and smuggled him out of his hospital bed and into a wheelchair. With him wrapped in blankets and his oxygen tank in tow, we went outside and stood in the rain. People shouted at us to come back inside, but he said, 'No, Deborah, don't. This is the last time I'll ever feel rain. Isn't it wonderful?' As I choked away the tears, I realised what an incredible lesson he was teaching me. That you can find positives even when it seems as though there is nothing to be grateful for.

I'm not saying you should look on the bright side whatever the circumstances, because sometimes things come along that are really shit, and to pretend otherwise is dishonest, or totally unrealistic. But I have always thought, and my experiences over the last few years have confirmed this for me, that how we see things is what matters, not necessarily what those 'things' are.

Before cancer, I thought I was grateful. I thought I took enough time to appreciate my children, my husband, my work and all the small things you barely notice but that bring happiness and add up to a lovely life. But I actually don't think that I truly did. I was pretty demanding of my life and had high expectations, and I didn't really appreciate the basic, little things at all. I think this was because I just assumed I had a future, but also, on top of that, I never stopped to consider that all of those little things I took for granted were the things that somebody less fortunate than me could only dream about.

Take how ill I was in the first few months of 2022. I literally had to learn how to stand up and walk again. Now, if I have a day when I can walk around, or a day when I can go outside and meet people and have a little bit of human connection, or, to be completely honest, another day when I don't die, I'm so grateful for it. I'm incredibly thankful, because I've met so many people over the last five years who didn't get that extra day. So many people who would have given anything for the opportunity to try to stand up again, or to look around and appreciate the beauty of nature, or to see their children grow just one more day older.

Gratitude is one of the things that helps get you through. It is a gift that you cling to when so much is being taken away. Before cancer, I never truly appreciated how lucky I am to have my parents and my husband and my kids in my life. I loved them, of course, but I didn't realise just how important they were until I understood that my time with them would be cut short. My mum has been by my side every step of the way – she has even had to feed me like I'm a baby again – and my sister has helped me to shower and wash my hair. My dad and brother have both been there for me throughout this terrible journey too. And I cannot stress how grateful I am for that.

My husband Seb is my utter rock, and together we seem to be able to squeeze each other's hands, swallow our tears and laugh instead. I'm more grateful for him since I've become ill than in the previous 15 years of our marriage. For the most part, it was a marriage filled with fun, but we were also working and bringing up our kids, just trying to do the best we could, with all of the everyday challenges that life throws at you. Since my diagnosis, he's had to adjust his whole life, not knowing what's around the corner with my health. He's had to work from home, and he's had to be both parents to our kids, organising everything in our lives. He's always been a wonderful father, but he's gone above and beyond to support us all. He knows our children are going to be without me at some point and he will have to step into that role. My illness has taken its toll on him, but I've also seen him

Gratitude is one of the things that helps get you through.

flourish as a person, and I am just so grateful to know that my kids will be in good hands when I'm not here.

One of the key challenges in my situation is that you don't want life to stop for everyone around you, just because it's stopped for you. Cancer, or any illness or significant life challenge, will very often drag everybody around you into it as well. And although in some ways you need and want that to happen, so that you have support and don't have to face your problems alone, it can lead to a situation where those problems become all-consuming. I think it was about three years after my diagnosis when I realised that I spent the majority of my time 'doing cancer' – my whole life was taken up by it. After that, we got to a much better place in our family where we didn't need to talk about and be immersed in cancer 24/7.

Especially if it's a long-term illness, you don't want people to look back and say, 'What did we do for five years? Did we just sit by a bedside?' I need my kids to be happy. Yes, they want to be with their mum. But I don't really want them to see me in pain; I want them to go out and enjoy life – amazing, wonderful, magical *life*. Just because I can't do stuff, especially since the beginning of 2022, doesn't mean that I want them to miss out.

Seb is half-French and he has family there, so he took the kids to visit them during the 2022 Easter break. They adore France, where they can run around outside with complete freedom, making bonfires and planting trees and playing with BB guns. Why should that stop for them? I don't feel like a burden, but I also need them to see life, because after I'm gone, I want them to still have a drive and desire for living. I don't want them to be consumed by the last five years. Which is why one of our strategies has been to get on with life despite everything. So, even at a stage when I probably needed people around me more than ever, I wanted them more than anything to go and have a fun holiday. It's what makes me happy, seeing pictures of them enjoying their life.

Before cancer, I also didn't truly realise how amazing my friends are. I have always been blessed to have good friends, but I never realised how far friendship can grow and how kind and generous people can be. For one thing, I think I had just assumed that people would talk to me about cancer all the time. That whenever I saw my friends, I would end up giving them an update about my situation, but other people have got stuff going on in their lives, and they don't always want to talk about how my cancer is progressing any more than I do. Instead, they showed their support in other ways – by having a natter on the phone, or taking me out for a drink, or going on a shopping spree. Then, when things got really tough, they stepped up and went further than you could possibly imagine to be the rocks that I needed.

I took the people in my life for granted, without a shadow of a doubt, and it makes me feel incredibly emotional to admit that. But I know that it's not just me. Lots of us do exactly the same thing, especially when we believe we have all the time in the world and the horizon seems long and uninterrupted. We go about our daily lives and are not truly grateful for the people we love. My diagnosis was in some ways a wake-up call. But I wish it hadn't taken this terrible experience to open my eyes. It's difficult when things are going well to take that step back, but, if you can, make yourself pause every now and again and think about what it would be like if the people you loved most in the world were taken away from you. I have no doubt that you, too, would have those feelings of gratitude that I have experienced.

After I'm gone, I want my kids to still have a drive and desire for living.

I'm also so incredibly grateful for basic human decency, generosity and selflessness, especially when it comes to the people who have taken care of me during the last five years of my illness. I think it's phenomenal what some people consider to be ordinary. In hospital, for example, I wouldn't want to clean up my mess let alone someone else's, but that's what the cleaning staff do without question. Or take the doctors who have kept me alive. According to them, they're just doing their jobs. To me, they're not just doing their jobs – they're performing miracles, and I'm in awe of them and relentlessly grateful that they have dedicated their lives to helping others.

Much of what I am grateful for comes down to the generosity of others. But trying to repay that generosity and being kind has also made me a better, happier and more positive person. My philosophy is: start small and start at home. For example, I'm gifted lots of beauty products, and I love passing them on, paying the generosity forward by matching kindness with kindness. It feels really, really good. Adding a smile to somebody else's day brings a smile to my day.

Once I shared a link via Instagram for a company I'd come across that sells scarves. I really liked what they were doing, because for every scarf they sold, they'd donate one to somebody who was currently undergoing cancer treatment. Because of my post, 150 scarves were bought, so the company sent me another 150 scarves, which I took round the Marsden for the other patients. I was so excited to do it, and it made me feel really happy to know that the repercussions of me doing something small and incredibly simple, like sharing a link to a company that I thought was doing something really nice, led to a little bit of kindness spreading even further.

I love it when people perform random acts of kindness. I'm often sent flowers by people who I don't really know and it truly brightens my day. And I think what makes this sort of thing even more impactful is that there are no ulterior motives behind it. These people don't expect anything from me in return – they just want to do something nice that will make someone else feel good. And when I gave out the scarves, I wasn't expecting anything back. Yes, it made me feel good to do it, but I wasn't motivated by that – my first thought was cheering up some of my fellow patients because it's rubbish being in hospital. A genuine act of kindness needs to be done with absolutely no expectation that you'll get anything back from it, because otherwise it changes the nature of it. It's a bit of a cliché, but it really is the thought that counts.

We have been bombarded with images and stories of war and corruption in recent years. As a result, it has become easy to lose sight of the fact that there are a lot of good people in the world, people who care about their communities and helping others. My advice is to look for the good. It's a choice to do so. No one is 100 per cent one thing or another –

Much of what I am grateful for comes down to the generosity of others.

the vast majority of people are not inherently good or bad. We are all flawed, so focus on the positives in people, and be thankful for those around you who give you life.

I'd argue that being grateful makes you a better person, but studies have been done that even show it makes you happier and healthier too. In fact, it's thought to be one of the most important factors when it comes to people's satisfaction with life – something I can personally vouch for wholeheartedly. It's partly because of the virtuous circle that gratitude creates. According to Alex Wood, who is a professor of psychological and behavioural science at the London School of Economics, 'People who feel more gratitude in life should be more likely to notice they have been helped, to respond appropriately, and to return the help at some future point.' But it doesn't end there: if the person who receives the help is grateful and decides to return the favour, a virtuous cycle is created. This in turn leads to better personal relationships, which, as we have seen, are so important in promoting and maintaining good mental and physical health.

Depending on our own personal circumstances, some of us naturally, and understandably, feel gratitude more easily than others. On top of this, there are times when all of us lose sight of the things that we are truly grateful for in life. If this is something you would like to explore, there are proven ways to integrate gratitude into our lives. For example, one study that investigated the impact of 'gratitude interventions' found that people who wrote a letter to someone meaningful in their lives to thank them for helping them and delivered it personally were happier and less depressed for up to a month afterwards. I think that's fascinating. Even more effective, however, was the gratitude journal. People who wrote down a list of three things they were thankful for every day for one week were happier and less depressed six months after performing the exercise. It was so successful that many of the participants incorporated the practice into their daily lives and felt all the better for it.

I have written lists of things I am grateful for at various points in my life, and I always found it incredibly beneficial. They included really simple things, like, 'Today I'm grateful because I'm seeing my friends and going to the cinema.' As my health deteriorated, I was grateful if I had a pain-free day, my blood markers were more positive or I was able to stay awake for a few more hours. Sometimes you have to aim for things that are achievable and take the wins you can get. If I was bitter about losing what I used to be able to do, I'd never be grateful for anything ever again.

Being ill has shown me that it is the basic things in life I most took for granted that I now miss the most: my house, being able to get into a car and drive somewhere, picking up my children from school, being able to walk, going outside and admiring the trees and breathing in the fresh air. I never understood the true value of being able to make it to one of my kids' school plays, for example. I was often too busy with work to attend. Then, in March 2022, the doctors at the Marsden moved mountains so that my drains could be taken out and I could go and see

'Expressing gratefulness during personal adversity like loss or chronic illness, as hard as that might be, can help you adjust, move on and perhaps begin anew. Although it may be challenging to celebrate your blessings at moments when they seem least apparent to you, it may be the most important thing you can do'

Sonja Lyubomirsky, *The How of Happiness*

my son Hugo in his school play. It meant the world to me, because I knew I would probably never get to see him performing again.

It's those little things that I took for granted or dismissed that are now the things in life that I crave more than anything. I have a beautiful common at the end of my road, and when I was stuck in a hospital room, I wanted so much

Sometimes you have to aim for things that are achievable and take the wins you can get.

to be strong enough to walk down to the common and sit and enjoy being in one of the places that I love most in the world. I used to run there every single day. I used to be able to leave my front door with my keys and seize whatever the day threw at me. I'd put on my running gear, even after I was diagnosed with cancer but was still well enough, and I'd shut the front door and decide where to go. Sometimes I'd take a wrong turn and end up at Tower Bridge or something, but it didn't matter. It's amazing when the sun is shining and you just feel utterly free. And now I can't even walk. I have had to readjust my expectations time and again, which in turn has allowed me to readjust what I'm grateful for.

I think the fact that I really want to live has made me so deeply grateful for the idea of living while I'm dying – of being grateful for every day that I am able to make new memories with my loved ones. Like the time, in May 2022, when Seb whisked me at the crack of dawn to the beautiful gardens of RHS Wisley in Surrey before the crowds arrived. I hadn't left the house for ten days, as I had been too weak, and while I then had to snooze for the rest of the day (in the sun like a cat!), I was so grateful for the reminder of the vibrant green life all around me. We all think we're going to live for ever and that life will be plain sailing. But we don't and it's not. Life can get tough, but then we can get tougher. Living in the face of death is the hardest thing I've ever done, but it has truly shown me the power of gratitude.

'A single act of kindness throws out roots in all directions, and the roots spring up and make new trees'

Amelia Earhart

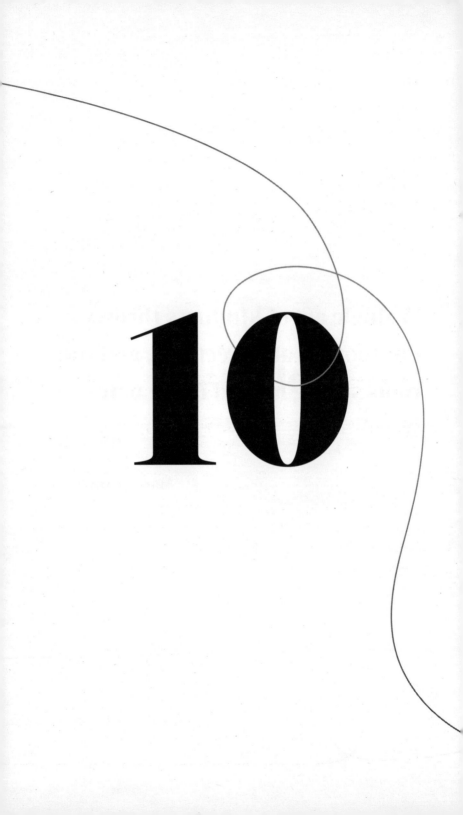

planting
seeds

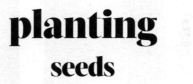

'Even if I knew that tomorrow the world would go to pieces, I would still plant my apple tree'

Martin Luther

I've planted so many seeds in my life, particularly during the last five years. Not actual seeds – I'm not wild about mud – but metaphorical ones. I've raised a son and a daughter and taught them life lessons early because I know I'm not going to be around when they're grown. I've educated people about cancer, I've run a marathon, I've fought for legislative change and I've stood up to bullies. I've talked for those who can't talk for themselves. And the reality is that I won't be around to see the fruits of all that labour. I won't live for as many years as I want, but I hope the work I've done and the love I've given and received will be around long after I am.

I never really thought of any of this as being part of my legacy until I started to look back at my life. For example, in five years of campaigning to raise awareness of bowel cancer, I never once stopped to think what my legacy would be or if it even mattered if I had a legacy or if one was important to me. Is it really important to any of us as we go about our day-to-day lives?

I've always had a message, which is to encourage conversation and debunk myths about bowel cancer so that fewer people have to suffer what I'm going through. I've worked as hard as I could to educate people about the disease. I've tried to frame the debate, talk about treatments,

I've worked as hard as I could to educate people about bowel cancer.

interview experts, and put a personal face on government cuts and figures about cancer and access to care. And I've wanted my cancer family to know how much I loved and cared for them. But I never thought about any of this as my legacy. I just thought it was my job and something to focus on and keep me going.

The same goes for whenever I think about myself as a daughter, sister, wife, mother and friend. I don't think about my legacy – I think about how I want my loved ones to remember me. I want them to picture me as this fun and vivacious person who they loved spending time with, even if I was a little bit all over the place at times and would never do the washing up. All I've ever wanted is for my kids and husband and family to love me and be proud of me.

I don't know how many of us go through life thinking about our legacies. Maybe it's a driving force for some people. But my hunch is that, for most people, it never really crosses their minds. And maybe it's better that way. I never knew how or when or why I might have touched somebody's life, but now, at the end of mine, I am receiving countless letters and cards from strangers, sometimes after they've arrived at my mum and dad's with just my name and no address on the envelopes, saying that I helped them in some small way. It is the most amazing thing. We never really know what impact we have on the people in our lives, and I had no idea when I started talking candidly about my situation that it would end up serving as inspiration for others. So, I feel hugely privileged to have seen that unknown legacy turn into a known one. Most people never have the privilege and honour of seeing the impact they have had, but the reality is that we touch people all the time, every day, even if we don't realise it.

It's happened to Seb too. He's received messages from people at work telling him how much he's helped them or positively impacted their lives and asking if there's anything they can do to repay him now that he is going through all of this with me, but, if it hadn't been for my illness, they probably wouldn't have ever told him. He's been grateful for the opportunity to learn that he's had a positive effect on people's lives, and so have I.

* * *

I always thought I could make a deal with the devil and things would turn out OK – in fact, I'm still in denial about the fact that I can't – so, as I've said, I never thought about what my legacy might be until my medical options ran out. It was only at that point when I suddenly felt I needed to think about what I was leaving behind. That's when my family and I set up the Bowelbabe Fund for Cancer Research UK and before I knew it I had a legacy. Despite initially aiming to raise £250,000, in just over two weeks we had raised more than £6.5 million! It was surreal and so far beyond what I ever could have imagined. All the money raised will be allocated to funding projects that I really care about, including clinical trials and research into personalised medicine that could result in new treatments for cancer patients and continued support to raise awareness of the disease. These funds will help so many more people benefit, like I have, from the amazing work of these causes in the years to come and maybe, just maybe, we can give one final 'f*** you' to cancer!

In my mind, I'd just been talking about poo for five years. And suddenly I go from that to being made a dame and meeting Prince William in my mum and dad's garden and being on the front pages of the newspapers. I didn't even recognise myself. I genuinely just thought I was talking about poo all this time. It's amazing, but you don't realise how big the repercussions of your small actions are until somebody stops and says, 'Hang on a moment. You've done pretty well.' And that can be a hard thing to grasp, because you're incredibly grateful, but it's not what you intended.

It's been like living in a dream. But it's not something that I ever aimed for. If I had aimed for it, I don't think it would feel as good as it does now. I am so grateful.

It's a bit like when I talked about kindness in the previous chapter. You don't do something for someone else with any expectation of reward or recognition. You do it because it's the right thing to do. If you do something with an expectation of recognition, it changes the whole act.

I feel hugely privileged to have seen that unknown legacy turn into a known one.

You might think that legacy is something you have to work towards knowingly or something that has to be achieved in your lifetime. Actually, your legacy is planting seeds that you will never see flower. Your legacy is knowing that you've done better for the next generation. Your legacy is having the rebellious hope that the actions you take today will create a better society tomorrow. Teaching taught me this. Teachers rarely know what our students will go on to achieve. All we can do is give them the tools and equipment, and hope that they can fly.

And we do that with our own children as well. We can't hold their hands every step of the way and tell them how to create their own legacies. We can only hope that we can instil the values in them that will make them want to go on and repeat the cycle and pay it forward.

'Don't judge each day by the harvest you reap but by the seeds that you plant'

Robert Louis Stevenson

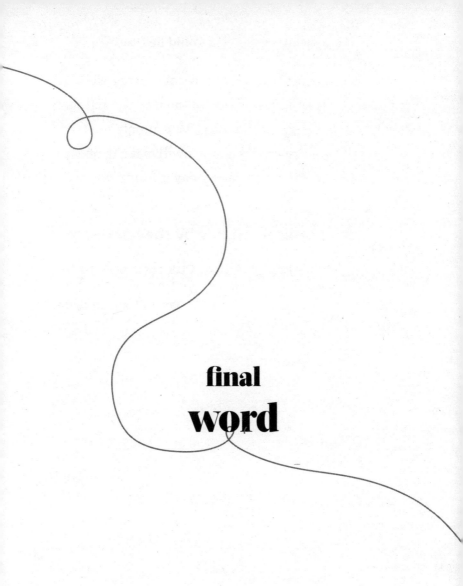

final
word

As I approach the end, my appreciation for the little things in life has only increased: walking from the kitchen into the garden and enjoying the sunshine; listening to the birds sing; having something to eat. You can get so caught up in stuff and take yourself so seriously, but when you get to this point in your life, the things that you might have worried about are brought into perspective. You realise that nothing else matters beyond the simple things and the love of your family and friends. You just want to be with them and tell them how much they mean to you.

After I moved to hospice care at my mum and dad's, I posted a picture of me sitting in the garden in the rain. It reminded me of my friend Simon who had cystic fibrosis. You never know when it will be the last time you're going to feel the rain on your face. You don't know whether, when you wake up in the morning, you will have the privilege of a full day. And yet we so often take the simple things for granted, like feeling the wind in our hair or the rain on our faces. I've never really liked the rain, but, sitting in the garden, I thought it might be the last time I'd ever feel it, and I wanted to embrace the experience, just like Simon had. You never know when it is going to be the last time you do something.

At the end of your life, you might think you would have all these grand plans – like going travelling and gallivanting here and there. But it's the simpler, more enduring things that blow you away. Like being told that a rose is being named in my honour – the Dame Deborah James Rose. I actually cried when I found out about it, because it was such a beautiful gift. Roses are my favourite flowers, and I hope this one will brighten everyone's smiles. It also brings me so much joy to know that the rose will be incorporated into a scheme that aims to get more vulnerable groups and people from underrepresented backgrounds involved in gardening. This variety can now be grown for ever, and maybe one day Eloise might even choose to have it in her wedding bouquet – a wonderful yet bittersweet thought.

Nothing else matters beyond the simple things and the love of your family and friends.

You have to savour life and enjoy the little things. Be grateful that you can simply move around. Take pleasure in being with your family. Enjoy your body. When all is said and done, these are what give me the most happiness.

When I was diagnosed, I looked at my husband and kids and thought, 'I can't die now.' I felt unsatisfied and thought, 'If I die now, there are too many things left hanging.' I don't feel like that any more. I've got to the end, and I regret that I won't be able to watch my wonderful children grow up, of course, but that's it. I don't feel bitter; I feel proud. I don't have any regrets about the people I've loved, or about unfinished business, or about the things I've done with my kids, or about the memories I've made. Living your life so that you have no regrets isn't easy, but I feel like that's what I've achieved.

People have said that I am showing how it is possible to have a good death, but the reality is I'm petrified. Inside I am so scared. I hate that it all has to end and that I have to leave behind the people I love so much. There's no amount of positivity that can overcome

You have to savour life and enjoy the little things.

that. All I can do is remind myself that my loved ones will be looked after once I'm gone, that they'll be OK. They're proud of me, and they love me, and they'll remember me in lots of different ways. And they'll always have a bit of my rebellious hope inside them.

When it comes down to it, that's the most important message I can pass on to you. I have found lots of different ways to help me cope with my illness, from learning the lessons that failure has taught me to laughing and feeling gratitude for the blessings in my life, but the thing that has got me through the most is my rebellious hope. And I know that if you, too, can keep a bit of hope, even when the dark times come, you will be able to overcome any challenge and live a life full of joy and contentment and happiness.

Resources

Further Reading

9 Things Successful People Do Differently by Heidi Grant Halvorson (Harvard Business Review Press, 2017)

Bounce: The Myth of Talent and the Power of Practice by Matthew Syed (Fourth Estate, 2011)

F*** You Cancer: How to Face the Big C, Live Your Life and Still Be Yourself by Deborah James (Vermilion, 2018)

Grit: Why Passion and Resilience Are the Secrets to Success by Angela Duckworth (Vermilion, 2017)

Handbook of Adult Resilience edited by John W. Reich, Alex J. Zautra and John Stuart Hall (Guilford Press, 2010)

The How of Happiness: A Practical Guide to Getting the Life You Want by Sonja Lyubomirsky (Piatkus, 2010)

Mindset: Changing the Way You Think to Fulfil Your Potential by Carol Dweck (Robinson, 2017)

Outliers: The Story of Success by Malcolm Gladwell (Penguin, 2009)

Positive Psychology in a Nutshell: The Science of Happiness by Ilona Boniwell (Open University Press, 2012)

Positive Psychology: The Scientific and Practical Explorations of Human Strengths by Shane J. Lopez, Jennifer Teramoto Pedrotti and Charles Richard Snyder (Sage Publishing, 2015)

Quiet: The Power of Introverts in a World That Can't Stop Talking by Susan Cain (Penguin, 2013)

Thinking, Fast and Slow by Daniel Kahneman (Penguin, 2012)

Websites

angeladuckworth.com

apa.org

bowelbabe.org

bowelcanceruk.org.uk

cancerresearchuk.org

hbr.org

positivepsychology.com

positivepsychology.org.uk

psychologytoday.com

sciencedirect.com

References

American Psychological Association, 1 Feb. 2020. Building your resilience, retrieved from https://www.apa.org/topics/resilience/building-your-resilience

American Psychological Association and Discovery Health Channel, n.d. The road to resilience, retrieved from https://www.uis.edu/sites/default/files/inline-images/the_road_to_resilience.pdf

Beckett, S., 2009. *Company/Ill Seen Ill Said/Worstward Ho/Stirrings Still*, Faber & Faber

Blume, J., 2015. *Tiger Eyes*, Macmillan Children's Books

Britzky, H., 6 Oct. 2020. A new Army field manual has tips for 'productive self-talk.' Here are some examples the service should add, *Task & Purpose*, retrieved from https://taskandpurpose.com/mandatory-fun/army-manual-productive-self-talk

Brooks, A. C., 23 Sep. 2021. The difference between hope and optimism, *The Atlantic*, retrieved from https://www.theatlantic.com/family/archive/2021/09/hope-optimism-happiness/620164/

Bryant, F. B. and Cvengros, J. A., 2004. Distinguishing hope and optimism: Two sides of a coin, or two separate coins? *Journal of Social and Clinical Psychology*, 23(2), pp. 273–302

Campaign to End Loneliness, n.d. Risk to health, retrieved

from https://www.campaigntoendloneliness.org/threat-to-health/

Carstensen, L. L., 2006. The influence of a sense of time on human development. *Science*, *312*(5782), pp. 1913–15.

Dholakla, U., 26 Feb. 2017. What's the difference between optimism and hope? *Psychology Today*, retrieved from https://www.psychologytoday.com/gb/blog/the-science-behind-behavior/201702/whats-the-difference-between-optimism-and-hope

Edmondson, A. C., Apr. 2011. Strategies for learning from failure, *Harvard Business Review*, retrieved from https://hbr.org/2011/04/strategies-for-learning-from-failure

Frank, A., 2012. *The Diary of a Young Girl*, Penguin

Frankl, V., 2004. *Man's Search for Meaning*, Rider

GOALBAND, n.d. Gail Matthews research summary, retrieved from http://www.goalband.co.uk/uploads/1/0/6/5/10653372/gail_matthews_research_summary.pdf

Haimovitz, K. and Dweck, C. S., 2016. Parents' views of failure predict children's fixed and growth intelligence mind-sets. *Psychological Science*, *27*(6), pp. 859–69

Hill, N., 2004. *Think and Grow Rich*, Vermilion

Levy, M., 2012. *If Only It Were True*, Versilio

Martin, R. A., Puhlik-Doris, P., Larsen, G., Gray, J. and Weir, K., 2003. Individual differences in uses of humor and their relation to psychological well-being: Development of the Humor Styles Questionnaire. *Journal of Research in Personality*, *37*(1), pp. 48–75

Morishima, T., Miyashiro, I., Inoue, N., Kitasaka, M., Akazawa, T., Higeno, A., Idota, A., Sato, A., Ohira, T., Sakon, M. and Matsuura, N., 2019. Effects of laughter therapy on quality of life in patients with cancer: An open-label, randomized controlled trial. *PloS One*, *14*(6), p. e0219065

Moskowitz, G. B. and Grant, H. (eds), 2009. *The Psychology of Goals*, Guilford Press

Osin, E., 7 Mar. 2010. Measuring balanced time perspective using Zimbardo Time Perspective Inventory (ZTPI), Positivepsychology.org.uk, retrieved from http://positivepsychology.org.uk/measuring-balanced-time-perspective-using-ztpi/

Roosevelt, E., 2012. *You Learn by Living: Eleven Keys for a More Fulfilling Life*, HarperPerennial

Winfrey, O., Sep. 2002. Dream big. *The Oprah Magazine*

Wood, A., Joseph, S. and Linley, A., 2007. Gratitude – Parent of all virtues. *The Psychologist*, *20*(1), pp. 18–21

Wood, A., Joseph, S. and Maltby, J., 2008. Gratitude uniquely predicts satisfaction with life: Incremental validity above the domains and facets of the five factor model. *Personality and Individual Differences*, *45*(1), pp. 49–54

Zimbardo, P. G., 2002. Just think about it: Time to take our time. *Psychology Today*, *35*(1), p. 62

Deborah dictated this love letter to Sebastien, Hugo and Eloise shortly before her death in June 2022.

I am currently sitting here next to the love of my life, Sebastien. I never quite knew if you could really have a love of your life, but I now know what the very core of unquestioned love is between two people.

I have always loved my husband. I fancied him from when I first met him, and I knew I would marry him after our third date. It was clear to me that, while he wasn't perfect, there was something about him that was right for me. He respected me, and he never let me walk all over him or wrap him around my little finger. He has always been and always will be the one person who can come and make everything better at 3am. He makes me feel safe. If I look across any room 18 years later, I still find him the most attractive man there. He had to mellow like a fine wine, because he has a stubborn side, which makes the three-year-old in me want to throw all my toys out of the pram. He loves a feisty debate and loves to joke – sometimes I just prefer a movie and a glass of wine.

When I look back at our relationship and marriage, I realise that it didn't just happen without work. The complexities of daily life sometimes got in the way. It's easy to forget that the person you love is still there in front of you when things are clouded by the annoyance of childcare logistics, money pressures and living like ships in the night. I wish I had learned at a young age that making time for your marriage to work should be as much a part of your timetable as going to the gym or cleaning your teeth. It's important that you don't allow the big arguments to build up, when all you really want is to forget about everything and cuddle the one person whom you love.

As cancer brings my life to an end, I feel this cruel realisation that I'm not fully able to be myself with the one person I have adored and needed in my life more than anyone else. I feel robbed of the freedom of a body without pain to kiss with, the freedom for us to make whimsical plans for our future and retirement together. Our goals and dreams have had to be adjusted week by week and day by day, depending on my cancer.

My husband has always been my rock. He holds me up when I can't hold myself and wipes away my tears. And yet I've wondered every day how it must have felt for him when the fairy-tale marriage he signed up for became a daily struggle to survive and fight for an extra moment of living. I've wondered how he's felt knowing he is about to become a widower. I've wondered how he'll remember me, and I've wondered if he will be OK.

* * *

To Hugo and Eloise, I can't even speak about you without crying. You are my world.

I've learned that there are many ways to parent – nothing is right or wrong as long as there is love. I've also learned that children are more resilient than we think.

There are mental snapshots of being a parent that will never leave you. But the beautifully etched memories that will come to you in your death are not necessarily the ones you might expect. One of my first is of Hugo when he was four days old. He was lying next to me in our double bed in our flat, and he was looking for my breast to feed on – he was yellow and had a big conehead. I remember looking at this little six-pound ball cradled against my tummy and thinking that it was only at this point that I had begun to understand what love was. I now look at that same fourteen-year-old boy, who still takes the time to cuddle up next to me on the sofa, and I would give anything to continue being able to protect him in the way I did when he was just four days old.

I believe in self-fulfilling prophecies, I believe in rebellious hope and I believe my children will be OK when I die. Because if I tell them they won't be, then they might not be. I want them to realise that life does not always go according to plan. You can make plans, and you can have goals, but you have to be prepared for the fact that sometimes life is more interesting when you go off-piste – so be brave. Take a chance and back yourself. Remember to be your number-one cheerleader. Don't leave the world and all it has to offer until retirement – experience it now. Learn to balance living in the now and being present in the moment with your plans for the future (although this may be the hardest lesson of all). Marry only for love. Buy a dog – I bought Winston at one of the lowest points in my life, and he has made me so happy. Nature and animals make me happy – apart from peacocks. It is only towards the end of my life that I have really started to appreciate nature.

Take time out. Relaxing isn't an indulgence; it's a form of refilling ourselves – none of us can drink from empty cups.

Each day, do things that make you happy – build them into your life and never criticise others for the things that make them happy.

Every day we awake not knowing if we will see the full 24 hours of the day, so as the sun comes up on a new day, we should feel blessed. We are given 86,400 seconds every day, and we each choose how to use them. It is only as they begin to slip away from us that we understand the value of each and every one of those seconds. So, my greatest advice to you is that you can do whatever you want with those seconds. You can use them however you want. The choice is yours, but the future belongs to those who believe in the beauty of their dreams. Do you believe in yours?